PISS OFF
(Literally)

D1521661

PISS OFF
(Literally)

Controlling Your Incontinence After Prostate Surgery

Laura McKaig PT, MSPT

PISS OFF (Literally): Controlling Your Incontinence After Prostate Surgery

Published in the United States of America with Kindle Direct Publishing

Editor   Kaitlin Cordova
Cover Designer   Russell Barr
Illustrators   Russell Barr, Pelvic Guru LLC
Photography   Carol Barr, Jason Barr, Cory Finley

ISBN-13#: 979-8-8539686-4-6
First edition: August 2023

Disclaimer: This book was written as a guide to help men through the recovery process after prostate removal or surgery. The information, exercises, and activities in this book are provided as a general guideline. It is not medical advice. It is not a personalized physical therapy plan of care. I cannot assess your situation, nor can I guarantee that the suggestions in this book will work for you. However, thousands of men have found them to be helpful in reducing or even eliminating their urinary leakage, urgency, or frequency problems. My hope is that you can also begin to see positive results as you read this book and apply what you've learned to your daily life.

ACKNOWLEDGEMENTS

A Special Thank You To:

My husband Darrel
who has lovingly supported me in this work

My healthcare colleagues and my Uncaged Clinician family
who encouraged me to write—and finish—this book

My wonderful clients
who have taught me so much about perseverance, resilience, and
overcoming challenges.
Thank you for entrusting your care to me.

Dr. Rachel Rubin and Dr. Tracy Sher
who motivated me to advocate for better post-cancer care.
This is my way of shouting it from the rooftops!

Friends, physicians, educators, and researchers
whose collaboration helped turn this idea into reality.

FORWARD

By Russell Barr

Book Cover Designer
Prostate Cancer Patient and Survivor

Hey, guys! That's me on the front cover pointing at you, using my typical "listen up" pose. The reason for it is that Laura McKaig has written things in this book that you really do need to hear. I know because I'm also a recent prostate cancer survivor and Laura is my physical therapist. Not to mention that in the process of designing the cover and working on the illustrations—I read the book. This book is one of a kind. With important content you won't find anywhere else.

When Laura asked me if I'd like to write this forward to her book, I was glad to accept. As long-time family friends, I couldn't have guessed that our lives would be as intertwined as they are today. If you had told me back then that Laura would be helping me navigate the aftermath of my own bout with prostate cancer, I'd have thought you were crazy.

Now, back to me pointing at you. When my prostate trouble began, I wished someone had pointed at me, and said, "Now, listen up! There's this book you need to read."

I had good advice and guidance about treatment options for the cancer, and realized that for me, surgery was the answer. (Being awake during the biopsy was weird, but I lived to tell the tale.) I had great confidence in the surgeon and am now healing well. He was pleased that I had a physical therapist to pick up where he left off.

While reading, expect to be challenged in your thinking and in your actions. But know that with those challenges comes sound advice and answers to questions you didn't even know you had. One example that jumped out at me has to do with breathing. I needed to be reminded that there are proper ways to breathe. No kidding. For instance, when I'm exerting myself physically, I need to breathe out—that holding my breath is a bad idea, especially if I want to keep from wetting my pants. There's a picture in Chapter 7 where I'm lifting a log. You can almost see me thinking, "Breathe out!"

Look, you already know that your routine is going to change. Please use this book to help you create realistic expectations as well as real encouragement that will be the cobblestones you feel under your feet, as you navigate the path ahead. There really is hope. That hope is hinged on real action toward regaining control sooner, rather than later! Let Laura help you along. And don't be surprised when you catch yourself saying, "Hey, I have this book you need to read..." while striking the "listen up pose."

INTRODUCTION

"WHY DO YOU DO THIS?" (My Story)

I'm not a medical doctor. I'm not a prostate cancer survivor. I am not the daughter, wife, or sister of a man with prostate cancer. So, why did I write a book about prostate cancer recovery? Why do I even care?

Here's why…

It all began when I started my training to become a pelvic floor therapist. I had restarted my physical therapy career after a 14-year break, and this time around I wanted to specialize and do something different. You don't learn this specialty in PT school. You need to take classes and do lots of continuing education. So, I took my first class. I was rather shocked by how much I did not know about this part of the body! I was not alone; most of the other therapists in the class were really surprised, too. We had no idea. I learned so much that weekend and gained a few skills to help people in this area.

This introductory course was geared toward women. You'll usually hear the term "women's health" rather than "pelvic health" or men's health. In this class, we learned about the pelvic floor muscles as they relate to the female anatomy. People with vulvas and vaginas and uteruses and all that. But we didn't learn the male version of the anatomy.

I clearly remember one part of the class discussion diverting to this topic of male pelvic floor issues.

That made me think: hmmm, would I treat men? Would I be okay with that? Comfortable with it? And what would my husband think about it? When I got home, I asked my husband that question, and we had a good talk about it.

I said, "If I decided to treat men, what would you think about that? Would that bother you?"

He paused for a bit, and then he asked me, "Well, are the men that you would be treating coming to you because they have a medical problem that is very distressing for them?"

I said, "Yes they would, they would have medical problems—incontinence, sexual dysfunction, or pain, things like that."

He said, "Okay. And would you have the professional skills and knowledge to treat them, and to address this medical problem?"

I replied, "Yes, I would."

And then he simply said, *"What's the problem then? Go help them."*

I tell you, that really meant a lot to me to get my husband's blessing for this. Yes, he does know what I do. And he fully supports the fact that I'm helping other guys who have problems with leakage, pain, or other issues "down there."

That was the first step.

The second step of this journey took a very unexpected turn when my dream job as a pelvic PT suddenly fell through. No warning, just a phone call from the clinic owner the week before I would start, saying that they changed their mind about hiring me. And I was left with nothing to fall back on.

I was devastated.

This was a very dark time for me. But sometimes the dark threads in our lives create the most beautiful tapestries. I didn't see it at the time, but a beautiful story was being woven from this experience.

Long story short, I ended up in a geriatric setting—which I said I would never ever EVER do.

Never Say Never.

I fell in love with it! I discovered how much I enjoy working with that age group. I stayed until changes at the facility caused my hours to drop dramatically. I found another job at a nursing home. The rehab manager there wanted somebody who could address the pelvic health issues of the residents in the nursing home. Nobody was doing it, but they were asking for it. My new boss told me, "Go. Do whatever you need to do. I'll support you."

And that was the start of my new focus in pelvic health. I began creating what was the first ever pelvic physical therapy program in a long-term care setting, at least in our area. I had the skills and knowledge that I needed, but it still felt like a daunting task. I figured things out as I went, hoping that it was good enough and that I could help those who were asking for it.

Then one day a gentleman approached me in the hallway, asking to start therapy for his incontinence. He was my very first male pelvic floor patient, and his name was "James." You'll get to read James' story in the first chapter. It's quite amazing, and I hope that you find encouragement in it. I actually think I learned more from James than what he learned from me!

That is how I got started with male pelvic health. I worked at the nursing home for several more years, then went on to start my own private practice. I decided that I wanted to offer pelvic floor physical therapy to men as well as women. It was kind of interesting, I got a little bit of flack for it. I had people who didn't quite understand it and would make comments like, "what, men have a pelvic floor?" Or my favorite weird comment, "so what do you DO with men?"

Male pelvic floor physical therapy is something I'm comfortable with now. I wasn't at first. You learn to be comfortable with things that were originally uncomfortable. Talking to a guy about how his penis works was really difficult at first. Giving the verbal cues to activate the right pelvic floor muscles in the right position for a man—that took me a while to feel comfortable saying that to a guy! Now I'm okay with it, and I've learned to add an element of fun into the treatment sessions.

Someone who comes in to see me after prostate surgery or cancer treatments might also feel the same unease and discomfort I used to feel. Talking about these very private things can be intimidating and even embarrassing. In my clinic, we honor that and respect that. We want every man to feel as comfortable and safe as he can through this part of his recovery journey.

So, there you have it. My journey into pelvic health (and specifically male pelvic health) took some major detours and has had multiple roadblocks along the way. It's not been an easy process, but I can tell you that it was 100% worth it. As this journey continues, I'm looking for new ways to help even more guys with the side effects that come from prostate cancer treatments. This book is one of those ways.

Why Do I Say "Clients" and Not "Patients"?

As you start reading this book, you might wonder why I refer to the people I work with as clients. Does it sound a bit strange? Here's why I made the change.

A few years ago, I started treating more and more people who had complex medical issues. They had been through the medical system for a long time, had been endlessly poked and prodded, and felt very out-of-control with the direction of their healthcare.

They also felt abandoned or let down once their medical treatment was finished. They still had physical problems but those were not getting addressed. Now they were in my clinic, and they had the chance to DO something about their pain, leakage, or other problems "down there," with my guidance. They could have much more control over how their Success

Plan was created and how they would reach the goals they set for themselves. We become a team; their input and participation are just as important as mine.

Here is what I told one of the first men to come to me after changing our verbiage from "patient" to "client":

"You're a client now, I figured you've been a patient for long enough."

He smiled and nodded, then said, "Thank you for that.

PROLOGUE

This Prologue is in honor of Caesar Blevins. He often went by the nickname "Big C." He was a big, tall man with a big personality, a big infectious smile, and a big heart. Caesar passed away on April 7, 2021, after a long battle with prostate cancer. I wrote this prologue the week after his death.

I first met Caesar in November 2019. I had heard about a group called The Prostate Network which helped cancer survivors. I wanted to learn more about it, so I just randomly showed up one time. I didn't know what to expect, and I wasn't sure how much I'd be welcome in this all-male group. What I experienced that evening blew me away. I'd never seen anything like it. Here were men helping other men walk a very difficult journey. Each person there had a chance to talk, share, ask questions.

The last person to speak was this guy named Caesar. He talked for quite a while. (It was obvious that he was quite a talker!) As I listened, I heard his story unfold, and saw how he used that story to give counsel, support, and comfort to guys who were grappling with the reality of cancer in their lives. I decided to join the cause to help prostate cancer survivors in my own unique way.

I didn't know Caesar for long and I didn't get to spend much time with him. But I'll tell you this—he was one special guy. I considered him a friend, a mentor, and a brother in Christ. And he sure left a legacy. A legacy of advocating and fighting for more funding for research, better access to screenings, and narrowing the gap of racial disparity in prostate cancer care for black men. He was a positive influence in his neighborhood, within the larger prostate cancer community, and among the legislators in Washington D.C.

He left a legacy of unwavering faith and trust in God. I think God gifted that man with a double portion of encouragement and optimism! Not the fake kind or just a positive-thinking attitude. This was truly the essence of his being. One way he expressed that was in his Facebook posts. He would post something every day. Every. Single. Day. Whether he was at work, at the gym, or in a hospital bed. As long as he was able, he would write words of encouragement to others. During the uncertain times of COVID and the terrible racial unrest that shook our country, I would always look forward to reading Caesar's posts. They were hopeful and thought-provoking. He could get his point across without using words of anger, judgment, or bitterness. I think his message had more impact that way.

He left a legacy of gentleness with strength. Or strength with gentleness. I never heard him yell at someone or insult them publicly. When a new guy came to the Prostate Network meetings, Caesar would ask them to tell their story, no matter how long it took. He provided a safe place for them to talk, ask questions, process stuff. Yet his gift for discernment meant he would call someone out if they started raising objections that were a smokescreen, giving excuses, or just complaining for the sake of complaining. Caesar was not one to tolerate any nonsense!

He also left the legacy of "Warrior On." And warrior on he did, until his last breath.

What comes to mind when you think of someone with Stage 4 cancer? Caesar was Stage 4 for nearly ten years. Ten years! I had learned about the physical effects of cancer in the body, but I didn't hear about its day-to-day impact on someone's life. Caesar's story gave me a greater level of understanding about this disease and how terrible it can be.

It's not "the good kind of cancer." It's not always slow growing, it can totally ravish one's body. This is the reality of prostate cancer for many men. Those ugly facts sometimes get glossed over. Yet Caesar never let that reality destroy his spirit. He always had an encouraging word, was always lifting others up, and kept his mind and his body as active as he could.

And that is a big reason why I'm doing this. Why I've joined the fight to get these guys the rehab that they deserve but are not getting after their cancer treatments.

Caesar Blevins touched so many lives because of his prostate cancer. There's a growing community, here in Kansas City and throughout the nation, that will continue his legacy. Doing all they can—all WE can—to stamp out prostate cancer, and to walk alongside those men who now live with this disease. Caesar wanted to make sure that no man walked this journey alone! Let's keep his legacy going.

"Teamwork Makes the Dream Work"
--Big C

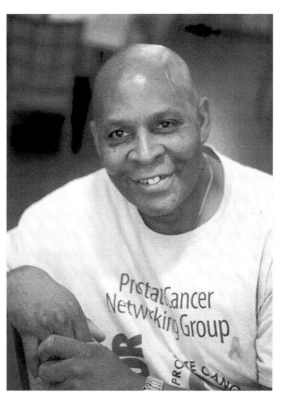

Caesar Blevins
Photo Credit: The Prostate Network

In Loving Memory of Caesar Blevins
May 24, 1957 - April 07, 2021

Table of Contents

CHAPTER 1

"HEY, WHAT ABOUT US MEN?"

James shoved a sheet of paper across the table, glaring at me. I could tell he was not pleased. What happened? Just a few days ago, James approached me in the hallway of the skilled nursing facility where I worked. A co-worker had told him about physical therapy for incontinence and suggested he talk with me. James was thrilled. He couldn't wait to get started! But today, he was staring me down from across the table with a scowl on his face. I looked down at the questionnaire that I had given him to complete before his evaluation. "You need to fix that" was all he said.

James had made a few obvious edits. I looked more closely. He had crossed out the words "woman," "women," and replaced them—in RED ink—with the words "MEN and women," "MAN or woman." It was then that I realized my huge oversight. The questionnaire I had given James was specifically for women with bladder leakage. At the time, I had not seen or treated any men with pelvic floor problems. So, I used the forms that I was familiar with, not realizing how biased they were.

I stared at the edited questionnaire for a moment longer, trying to hide my embarrassment. James's glare began to soften. "You know, Laura, these aren't just women's problems. Now why do you call it women's health, when we men have issues too? I'm feeling left out here, Laura."

Indeed, he was left out. James had come to our skilled nursing facility to recover from prostate cancer treatments. His medical needs were being cared for, except for the one thing that bothered him the most: his loss of bladder control. Nothing much was being done about it except giving him adult diapers to wear. James was a proud man and a veteran, and he found this humiliating. The only help he got from the urologist was a short paragraph about Kegel exercises in his hospital discharge papers. He had tried the Kegels the best way he could, but they weren't working.

Now James was not a guy who was content to "wait and see" if things got better. He started asking around when he arrived at the rehab center. Was there anyone there who could help him with his incontinence? Give him something he can actually DO about it himself? He was told that there was a "women's health specialist" on staff who might be able to help. (You can guess what he thought about that title!) But he was determined to find a solution. He found me in the hallway outside the therapy gym, and we talked. I told him that I thought pelvic floor physical therapy would help with his bladder problems. He brought the idea to his urologist who gave him the okay to start.

James was dealing with quite a few pelvic floor-related problems, including:

- Urinary frequency: He was getting up every 20 minutes at night to use the bathroom. He couldn't stand that. To make things worse, when he got up, even to use the bedside urinal, he would get dizzy. His dizziness greatly increased the risk of him falling and injuring himself.
- Urinary urgency: He couldn't hold it long enough to make it to the bathroom in time. This also increased his fall risk as he tried to rush to the bathroom.

- Pelvic floor muscle weakness: His pelvic floor muscles were very fatigued and weakened and didn't have the strength to maintain continence.
- Rectal and perineal pain from his cancer treatments: He was unable to sit comfortably in his wheelchair.

James was also very anxious about an upcoming event: his daughter was getting married in a couple of months, and he wanted to be there to walk her down the aisle. How is that possible, he thought?

In the weeks that followed, James taught me about pelvic floor dysfunction from a man's perspective. Here's what I learned:

- how distressing it is to men when they have problems with peeing
- how limited resources are for men regarding pelvic health
- the reality of how prostate cancer treatments can affect the pelvic floor
- how to use creativity and resourcefulness in solving his problems

We started his pelvic floor therapy. I only knew the basics at the time, had no prior experience working with prostate cancer, and was figuring things out as I went. I used some of the techniques and strategies that you will read about in this book. James learned not only how to strengthen his pelvic floor, he also learned how to suppress that strong urge and how to creatively use swim noodles to provide relief from sitting pain!

Despite my rookie status as a pelvic floor therapist, James got better. He was so thankful that there was someone willing to take him seriously, willing to listen to him and to honor and respect what he had to say. This is a very intimate area, the pelvic floor; it's hard to talk about it. He was very grateful to learn that he could actually do something about his problem. He worked hard, diligently participating in the pelvic floor therapy sessions for about eight weeks. He had a lot of medical issues going on which made things extra challenging. However, James made amazing progress.

When he was ready to return home,

- His daytime urinary frequency was nearly normal. He was only getting up 3 times at night instead of 18 times!
- He had gained sufficient pelvic floor strength to prevent urine leakage.
- He had learned how to "hold back the tide" when the urge hit. He could make it to the bathroom more calmly and in control with no accidents.
- He could sit comfortably in his wheelchair without pain.

He got to a point where he thought his bladder control was actually better than before he was diagnosed with prostate cancer! That amazed me. James also reached his ultimate goal. He was able to walk his daughter down the aisle at her wedding, with confidence. I was thrilled to hear that. This was life-changing for him.

James even wrote me a letter and gave me permission to share his story. He said, "Laura, whenever I go into the VA Clinic, and I go to the urologist office, I tell all the men in the waiting room about you." He was so excited that he was getting better, and he wanted to share that with other men who had similar problems, so that they could find help as well.

James was equally inspiring to me. Seeing the impact that this therapy had on his life, I wanted to help other veterans. Four years later, I finally became credentialed with the Veterans Association and am now providing help and hope (with a much better skillset!) to our veterans with prostate cancer. It is an honor to serve them in this way.

CHAPTER 2

"NO. NOTHING."

PISS OFF (Literally)

Did you notice the blank page? Yes, it is there intentionally. It is there to symbolize the lack of options given to men for their prostate cancer recovery.

If it surprised you to find out how little is available for men in general, the gap is even wider when it comes to men recovering from prostate cancer treatments.

I was on a phone consultation with José, a retired businessman living in Phoenix, Arizona. He called at the suggestion of his wife. José was diagnosed with prostate cancer seven years ago and chose robotic prostatectomy as his treatment. Like many men, he still suffers from lingering side effects: erectile dysfunction and incontinence.

We talked about his recovery experience after the surgery. He stated that in Phoenix there's lots of sexual wellness information available, yet nothing that addressed his specific problem. He had gone to his cancer center and was given a vacuum pump to help with erections. It did nothing for him. I asked him if anyone there had suggested pelvic floor physical therapy as an option. He quickly interrupted:

"NO! No. No option. Nothing mentioned."

I paused to soak that in a bit more. As José continued, his tone changed to frustration and a bit of anger. "This cancer center is always emphasizing how great they are, but they're not so great with helping you after the surgery or treatments are finished. They got what they wanted. Now, I have to deal with what's left."

(By the way, I often hear the same thing from other cancer survivors, about other cancer centers.)

Why is that so common? I won't try to explain why, defend, or rationalize. These cancer specialists are great at what they do. They save many lives, and for that we are grateful. Post-cancer care is not their specialty.

Let's look at the most common options given to these men.

"Wait and see" approach. Men are often told to wait for bladder control to come back on its own. "These things take time," they are told. And that's it. Why do I have a problem with this?

1. You may have already tried this "wait and see" approach with your prostate cancer. You may not be too thrilled to do another round of waiting.

2. Do you really want to just wait? It's true; studies show that with or without pelvic physical therapy intervention, continence control will often return on its own after about 12 months.[1] But do you really want to wait that long? Do you really want to buy Depends or pads every week for up to 52 weeks, putting up with wet pants, dealing with the smell, and avoiding the gym or golf course for that long?

Kegels. The extent of "pelvic floor therapy" offered to most men here in the U.S. is often just being told to "do Kegels" and that's it. That may work for some men, but for most, it is far from enough. Rarely is there any one-on-one instruction or guidance in how to do them correctly. (We will go over this in more detail in Chapters 7 and 8.)

Surgery. If moderate to severe incontinence persists, there are some surgical options which can help. The two most common are male bladder sling and AUS (artificial urinary sphincter). It is beyond the scope of this book to discuss each surgery in detail. The point is this: too often, men are not even given the option of trying pelvic floor physical therapy or any sort

---

[1] Filocamo, Maria Teresa et al. "Effectiveness of early pelvic floor rehabilitation treatment for post-prostatectomy incontinence." *European Urology* 48, no. 5 (2005): 734-738.

of pelvic muscle retraining before considering surgery. Could yet another surgery be avoided if they had pelvic PT first?

Online resources. I've heard from many prostate cancer survivors, and from men in general, that there are very few pelvic health resources available to them online. You would think that doing a Google search would turn up something, but often guys come up empty-handed. Or they find resources for their incontinence, but they're obviously geared toward women. As one frustrated guy said, "All I'm finding out there for resources is either pink or has lady bits on it!"

Bridging the Mile-Wide Gap

"The knowledge gap on physical therapy for prostate cancer patients is so large, every little bit we do will go miles."

They didn't know I was coming. I randomly showed up one evening to a meeting of a local prostate cancer support group. I wondered how I would be received, being the only female attending an all-male gathering. We had a funny mistaken identity at first, and I reassured them that I was not the speaker for the evening! I was not there to pitch physical therapy nor to talk about myself. I was there to listen and to learn how I could better help my prostate cancer clients. And learn I did. The group was founded by two guys named Steve and Caesar. Both are prostate cancer survivors; they started this group as a practical way to help other men with this diagnosis. I had never seen anything quite like it. And I heard things that I had not heard in any of my training or education classes about prostate cancer.

Here were my takeaways from that first night:

- Prostate Cancer is more common than I thought. One in six men will get prostate cancer. The ratio is even higher for black men and veterans.
- Men don't talk about it.
- Men don't tell their doctors about the side effects like erectile dysfunction and incontinence that they may be experiencing.
- The two main problems they want solved are incontinence and erectile dysfunction.
- They are not told about nonsurgical options for treatment of these problems.
- They are not given ANY education to prepare before surgery (prehab) and given NO recovery information after surgery or treatment.
- There IS no cancer survivor plan in place for these guys.

After the meeting, I talked with Steve. He was surprised to learn how much pelvic physical therapy could help. Surprised that after years of leading this group, he didn't really know much about it, and very few of the guys had gotten referred to PT after their surgery. He wanted to learn more. We decided to meet to talk further. Could we somehow combine our efforts to help these guys even more?

I learned more of Steve and Caesar's passion for helping support men through their journey with prostate cancer. I saw his desire to help more men bridge that gap between cancer treatment and living a fulfilling life after the treatment is over. He was learning how pelvic physical therapy could be one way to help bridge that gap.

"The knowledge gap on physical therapy for prostate cancer patients is so large, every little bit we do will go miles," Steve told me.

How could we accomplish this working together? By giving men more resources about pelvic physical therapy—what it is, how it can help them. And by educating them in self-advocacy.

The longer I'm doing this work, the more I think that men may be the most underserved when it comes to pelvic health awareness. As Steve mentioned, the knowledge gap is huge, for patients as well as for physicians.

I don't think that doctors (urologists, oncologists, general practice doctors) are intentionally hiding this from their male patients.

It's not that they're trying to hold a corner of the market, or they don't want to refer to physical therapy. They just don't know about it, it's not part of their training. Because of that, physical therapy is not a top-of-mind option for them.

The situation is slowly improving, but most men still are left to find resources on their own. Just because the doctors have no options to give you does not mean there are no options, it just means maybe they haven't pointed you to the right solution.

One solution is pelvic floor physical therapy. There are a lot of us around the country, and most of us are networked together. Maybe you bought this book to find out how you can help your dad, your brother, or your old platoon buddy. If you can find one pelvic floor PT to talk to, that one can usually find someone in the part of the country you need.

Another solution in narrowing the gap between cancer care and a fulfilling life is for men to share their stories. Stories of their journey with prostate cancer, and how they found help for these side effects. Men are very encouraged when they hear other men saying, I sure had a hard time finding this kind of help, but it was worth the time and effort. No man should have to go through this kind of journey alone.

Start talking about it. Help us bridge this mile-wide gap, one person at a time.

PISS OFF (Literally)

CHAPTER 3

THE "WHAT THE HELL!" MOMENT

That's what Gerard calls his experience post-surgery.

"I'll never forget what it was like when they pulled the catheter out after my prostatectomy. I was shocked at how much leakage there was! It was uncontrolled flooding. I had asked my medical team beforehand if it was common to have severe incontinence post-surgery. They said, 'Oh, no, that almost never happens. That won't be a problem.' Well, it was a problem. A big one. The nurse then gave me an absorbent brief to put on and said, 'Okay, you're good to go!' And they sent me home. That was all. I couldn't believe it. I thought, What the hell is happening…am I going to be like this the rest of my life? This was NOT part of the plan!"

Gerard did not have a plan because he didn't think he needed one. He found out otherwise. It took him three months of searching on his own before he found help that radically transformed his symptoms, his work performance, and gave him hope. He is sharing his story because he doesn't want other guys to go through what he did.

Gerard learned a valuable lesson: knowledge is power. Knowing what to expect can go a long way in helping you get through your surgery and recovery with a bit more reassurance, confidence, and a better sense of control.

Preparing for Your Surgery

What can you do to prepare yourself, and avoid your own "What the Hell" experience? Here's a few tips from pelvic health specialists, physicians, and fellow prostate cancer survivors:

1. Get information!

Find out about what to expect regarding the surgery, recovery, and possible side effects. Write it down so you can refer to it later; it's doubtful that you'll remember everything you need to know. Get a second opinion if what you're being told just doesn't sound right.

2. Make a Game Plan

Have a pre-surgery checklist ready. You can find one in the Recovery Toolkit at the end of the book.

- What do you need to know before your surgery?
- Who do you need to talk with?
- What problems might you have after surgery?
- How are you going to address these problems? What options are available?
- Where will you get support?
- Where will your caregiver get support?

If these questions left you with more questions, then keep reading. We'll go into more details in the next section.

3. Prehab!

"When you are going to have knee surgery, you usually get sent to physical therapy to strengthen your muscles beforehand. If we get PT to rehab our knee, why don't we get it to rehab our penis and bladder?"
—Steve, prostate cancer survivor

Want that incontinence to go away sooner than later? If you answered Yes, then the answer is to get your pelvic floor muscles in the best shape possible BEFORE your surgery. We call that "prehab." If you know someone who has had knee replacement surgery, often they do a short course of physical therapy beforehand to get their leg and hip muscles stronger and ready for the surgery and the rehab that follows.

If prehab works for knee surgery, would it also work for prostate surgery? Yes! The latest studies show that prehab reduces recovery time and makes the pelvic floor retraining process easier and more effective after prostatectomy, with faster results. Starting some basic pelvic floor training five weeks prior to surgery is ideal. We will discuss what this looks like over the next few chapters.[2,3]

---

[2] Milios, Joanne E., Timothy R. Ackland, and Daniel J. Green. "Pelvic floor muscle training in radical prostatectomy: a randomized controlled trial of the impacts on pelvic floor muscle function and urinary incontinence." *BMC Urology* 19, no. 1 (2019): 1-10.

[3] Mungovan, Sean F. et al. "Preoperative exercise interventions to optimize continence outcomes following radical prostatectomy." *Nature Reviews Urology* 18, no. 5 (2021): 259-281.

What You Might Want to Know

"I wish I had known this before my surgery."
—said by hundreds of survivors

I've heard from so many prostate cancer survivors that they wish they had been given more information before their surgery. It wouldn't change the outcome, but it would at least give them more peace of mind, less anxiety, and the hope that "this too shall pass." It can also give them some sense of control, knowing that they CAN do something about the side effects that may happen after surgery.

The problem is that you might not know what questions you need to ask at your surgical consult or follow-up visits. Just knowing that you have cancer is overwhelming. If you don't know what questions to ask, the doctor won't know which questions to answer or anticipate. That's when miscommunication or lack of communication can happen.

Would you like to go to your consult or follow-up visit more prepared but don't know what to say? Here's a list of some of the more common questions that men have regarding urinary control:

- What the heck does the prostate do, anyway?
- Why am I leaking like a sieve after the surgery?
- Can robotic surgery prevent incontinence as a side effect?

You may think of additional questions. Let's answer these three, starting with:

1. What does the prostate do?
The prostate is a gland located between the bladder and the pelvic floor (more on those in the next chapter). Its main function is to produce some of the fluid in semen, the product of ejaculation.

The prostate also supports the bladder neck, at the bottom part of the bladder. The urethra (aka "pee hole") passes right through the prostate like the core of an apple. The prostate tissue helps to provide structural support for the urethra.

Illustration 3.1 gives you a frontal view of where the prostate, bladder, and urethra are inside your body.

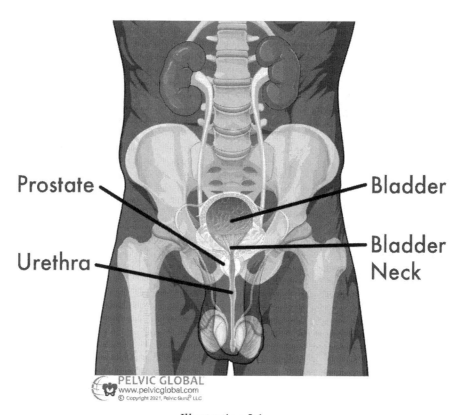

Illustration 3.1

Image used with permission from Pelvic Guru®, LLC www.pelvicglobal.com

The prostate is also close neighbors with an important muscle, the internal urethral sphincter. This internal sphincter muscle sits right between the bladder neck and the prostate. Although it is a circular muscle, it acts like a valve, closing to keep urine in the bladder and opening to let urine out. The internal urinary sphincter is the first of two such "valves" (the second valve is the external urinary sphincter, located further down the urethra).

2. Why am I leaking so much urine after prostate removal?

Why are the bladder neck and the internal urinary sphincter important to know about? Here's why: After the prostate is removed, the bladder neck is stretched down and is attached to the end of the remaining urethra. This process either removes the internal urethral sphincter or renders it non-functional.

Earlier in this chapter, I mentioned that you have two sphincter muscles, circle-shaped muscles that open and close to keep in urine or let it out at the right time. One is under your control (external sphincter), one is not (internal sphincter). With removal of the internal sphincter, your two-valve system now has only one valve, making it more difficult to control urine flow. That's one reason many men feel they leak like a sieve right after prostatectomy.

Your external sphincter and other pelvic floor muscles must assume a "new identity" now that the prostate and internal sphincter are gone. They can no longer rely on the prostate to play a major role in bladder control. They need to work in a different way. These muscles need RETRAINING, not just strengthening. This is one reason why some men struggle with incontinence for months or years after surgery. And why pelvic floor retraining can help.

<u>3. Does robotic surgery eliminate side effects?</u>

The short answer: No, robotic surgery does not guarantee zero side effects.

You may have heard that having the robotic procedure shields you from the side effects of incontinence.

There are many advantages to this kind of surgery, such as smaller incisions, less blood loss, shorter hospital stay, less pain, and faster recovery time.

However, it does not eliminate the risk of side effects. There's still the risk of leakage. Studies have shown that the single most important factor in your surgery success is the skill of the surgeon, not the specific surgical method.[4]

"Knowing what to expect helped lower my anxiety about the surgery. It also gave me confidence that, should problems arise, I'll know how to handle them so that they don't control my life. That gives me so much relief!"
—"Devon," prostate cancer patient and survivor

After Surgery: First Steps

You've just had your surgery. All the things you may have learned at the doctor's office are forgotten as you deal with "NOW what do I do?"

Of course, you should follow your surgeon's post-operative instructions.

Beyond that, here's a few simple tips and tricks that other men have found helpful when they first return home.

---

[4] Chang, Peter et al. "Prospective multicenter comparison of open and robotic radical prostatectomy: The PROST-QA/RP2 Consortium." *The Journal of Urology* 207, no. 1 (2022): 127-136.

Buy pads or briefs

You will need them at first as your body starts to recover. There's quite a selection nowadays. Even if your surgeon told you that you'd be fine, have some on hand just in case you aren't. You don't want to get caught without any if you really need them!

You would think that shopping for incontinence briefs or pads would be easy, right? Wrong; many guys have told me that it can be an overwhelming experience. They find different brands and different thicknesses of briefs, pads, guards, shields…guards and shields?! What the heck are those?? No worries: more detail on how to select briefs, pads or guards is in Chapter 8. For now, just focus on getting one or two packages of briefs and/or maximum absorbency pads.

Be sure you get pads for bladder leakage, not feminine pads. Menstrual pads are not made to absorb urine. Also note that men need more absorption near the front of the brief or pad, and women's pads are not designed that way.

You can order pads or briefs online; for some men this is a great and discreet option. Many men prefer the Tena brand that is currently available. Some companies will even provide you with free samples. It wouldn't hurt to ask!

Puppy pads!

Yes, puppy training pads. These are a great option to put on your bed at night or in your chair if you're concerned about excessive leakage. You can find them anywhere. They are much cheaper than adult incontinence pads (also known as chucks). Less embarrassing, too—people will just think you're training a puppy when you're in the store checkout line.

Begin Bladder Retraining Basics

You may be thinking, what does "bladder retraining" mean exactly? Am I going to teach my bladder to lift weights or something? No, it's not that kind of retraining. It means that you can teach your bladder to behave in a certain way. In this case, to behave more like it should. In the next chapter, we'll help you establish a baseline for your bladder function.

For now, here are some tips to encourage good bladder habits the first 4-6 weeks after surgery:

Decrease caffeine intake
Limit yourself to 1 drink/day MAXIMIM.
That includes coffee, tea, green tea, and sodas.

Increase water intake
Drink it throughout the day, not just in the morning or at night.
How much water intake is adequate? In general, half your body weight in ounces, more if you are doing strenuous activity/exercise.

Decrease fluids at nighttime
Begin drinking less fluid approximately 2-3 hours before bedtime.
This can help reduce nighttime leakage or urinary urgency

NO alcohol for the first 4-6 weeks!
Here's why: 1) Alcohol doubles urine production and 2) it relaxes your muscles—including pelvic floor muscles—making it harder to keep your urethra closed.

Avoid or minimize common bladder irritants
These can include alcohol, caffeine, carbonated beverages, citrus, MSG, spicy foods, tomatoes.

Schedule your times to urinate
Go use the toilet at set times, whether you feel the urge or not.
You can start with urinating, or voiding, every hour. This is also called timed voiding. It helps with the bladder retraining process.

Then, gradually increase your voiding time
Start increasing the time in between voids, in 10-15 minute increments, from every hour to every 2 hours, and finally to every 3-4 hours.

This allows the bladder muscle to get used to expanding normally again and holding a normal volume of urine.[5]

Be Aware of What to Expect as You Recover

Not knowing what to expect for recovery can be really stressful when you have little to no bladder control. Here is a general guide of how most men progress with their urinary control. You might expect the following changes, with estimated time frames (your time frame may vary):

- First 1-3 Weeks: you leak day and night when you first come home
- 3-6 Weeks: you become dry at night first but are still leaking during the day
- 4-6 Weeks: most of your leakage occurs when changing positions, such as sitting to standing, or when bending forward.
- 6 Weeks to 6 Months: you still leak with certain activities, but the leakage occurs less often or is less in volume
- 10-12+ Weeks: post-void dribble is still common even after the daytime leakage subsides
- 12+ Weeks: late afternoon/evening leakage is often the last to resolve
- 6-12 Months: leakage may get worse or recur when doing strenuous activity or when drinking alcohol

---

[5] Claire C. Yang and Gerald W. Timm. "William E. Bradley and his contributions to urology." *The Journal of Urology* 179, no. 5 (2008): 1700-1703.

<u>When Can You Start Basic Pelvic Floor Strengthening?</u>

First, consult with your surgeon to get the okay to start. Sometimes surgical or other medical issues may require that you delay starting these exercises. In general, however, you should wait until your catheter is out before starting any pelvic floor strengthening. Attempting pelvic floor exercises with a catheter still in could cause further irritation to the bladder.

PISS OFF (Literally)

.

CHAPTER 4

PELVIC FLOOR, PISTONS, PEEING: What's The Connection?

WHAT IS THE PELVIC FLOOR?

I've already been talking about the pelvic floor. You may have thought this is only something that women deal with. However, men have a pelvic floor too. When your pelvic floor is in good working order, you don't need to think about it much at all.

So what exactly is the pelvic floor? And why is it important in solving your leakage problem after prostate surgery or removal?

The area between your scrotum and anus (called your perineum) is made of muscle and is part of the pelvic floor. The pelvic floor is made up of about 20 different muscles, in 3 layers. You can find it on yourself. It goes from your pubic bone in front (above the base of your penis), down and back to attach to the tailbone, or coccyx. It also attaches to each of your sit bones (or "butt bones"). See Illustration 4.1

It resembles a hammock from front to back, and from side to side. In a way, it's like a floor. A floor made of muscles. A "pelvic floor."

YOUR PELVIC FLOOR
(Bird's Eye View)

Spine & Tailbone

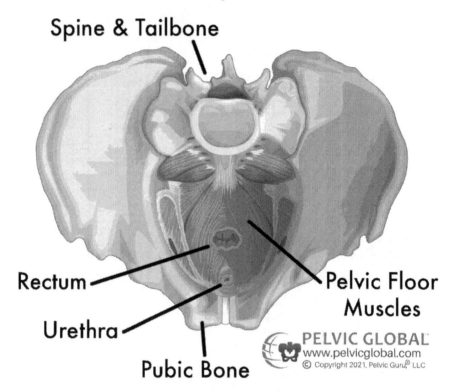

Rectum

Urethra

Pubic Bone

Pelvic Floor Muscles

PELVIC GLOBAL
www.pelvicglobal.com
© Copyright 2021, Pelvic Guru® LLC

Illustration 4.1

Image used with permission from Pelvic Guru®, LLC www.pelvicglobal.com

PELVIC FLOOR, PISTONS, PEEING: What's The Connection?

The male pelvic floor has 4 important functions. I call them the 4 S's:

1) Support. The deeper layer supports the abdominal and the pelvic organs (bladder, prostate, colon).
2) Stabilize. It helps to stabilize your spine as well as your pelvis and your trunk, so that your arms and legs can move and lift and do what they need to do.
3) Sphincter control. The urinary and anal sphincter muscles are part of the pelvic floor. They let you hold in your pee, your poop, or your gas when you want to hold it in and let it out when you want to let it out. The muscles in the front layer also help with urinary control.
4) Sex. Yessir, the pelvic floor has a really important role in sexual function as well! The muscles toward the front are specially designed to help achieve erection and ejaculation.

Your pelvic floor is amazingly complex! Not only do the muscles have different roles, but the muscle fibers themselves have different functions. Your pelvic floor muscles are made up of two kinds of muscle fibers, called "slow twitch" and "fast twitch" fibers. These different muscle fibers have different purposes.

Illustration 4.2 is a graphic description of your two pelvic floor muscle fibers (pun intended).

Fast Twitch vs Slow Twitch Muscle Fibers

Fiber Type	SLOW TWITCH	FAST TWITCH
Where?	In back, closer to rectum	In front, closer to penis & scrotum
Designed For:	Endurance, Stability	Power & Speed
Is Like A:	Marathon Runner	Sprinter
Most Active During:	Prolonged Standing, Walking	Coughing Sneezing Lifting

Illustration 4.2

Why is this information important to you? Because these muscle fibers have different retraining needs!

A marathon runner would not train the same way as a sprinter. In the same way, you need to train your slow twitch muscle fibers differently than you do your fast twitch muscle fibers.

New research shows that this difference is very important and can lead to better results for bladder control.[6] You'll learn more about this in Chapter 11.

THE PELVIC CONNECTION

When you are trying to regain your bladder control, bowel control, or sexual function, you need to include the rest of the body in the process. The pelvic floor does not work in isolation.

What is this Pelvic Connection? And how is it connected to the rest of the body?

I'll use two of my favorite analogies to explain:

Soda Can Analogy

Why would I use a soda can to talk about the pelvic floor? Here's why: your pelvic floor is considered the "floor" of your core. Take a look at the illustration. You notice the soda can has a top, a bottom, and sides. Let's say the top of the soda can is our diaphragm, which is our big breathing muscle. The bottom of the soda can is the pelvic floor. The front represents our deepest layer abdominal muscles, and the back of the can is the little muscles in between each bone of our spine, called multifidus (plural multifidi).

Illustrations 4.3, 4.4

---

[6] Milios, Joanne E., Timothy R. Ackland, and Daniel J. Green. "Pelvic floor muscle training in radical prostatectomy: a randomized controlled trial of the impacts on pelvic floor muscle function and urinary incontinence." *BMC Urology* 19, no. 1 (2019): 1-10.

SODA CAN ANALOGY

Top = Diaphragm

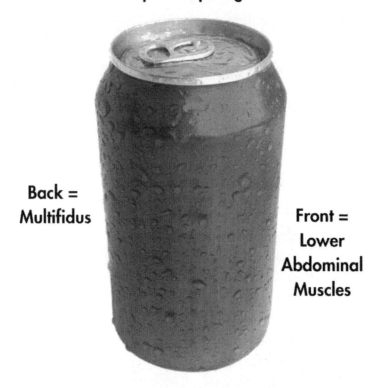

Back =
Multifidus

Front =
Lower
Abdominal
Muscles

Bottom = Pelvic Floor Muscles

Illustration 4.3

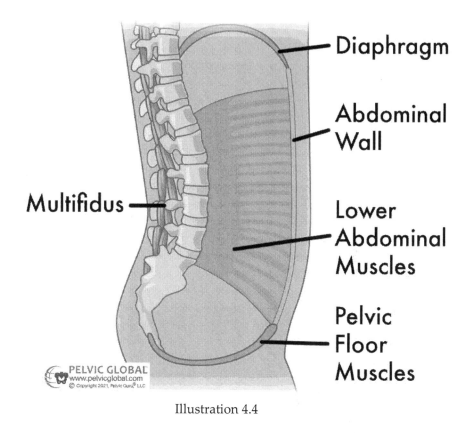

Illustration 4.4

Image used with permission from Pelvic Guru®, LLC www.pelvicglobal.com

Just like the soda can, you really can't take one of those parts and work it just by itself. Our bodies are not made that way. There are connections with joints, with connective tissue and with muscle that connect our diaphragm with our pelvic floor, and that connect our pelvic floor with our abdomen and our low back. These muscle groups were made to work as a team.

When you have incontinence or pain, often the muscles are not working together and they're not doing their job. What you need to do is retrain them in a way that helps them work together again as a team. This involves more than just strengthening the pelvic floor. A "teamwork" approach will get your bladder control back more quickly and more effectively. I'll explain more about that in Chapter 8.

Piston Analogy

I also use a piston analogy to talk about the pelvic floor connection with the diaphragm muscle. You may be familiar with what a piston is and how it works. (Illustration 4.5)

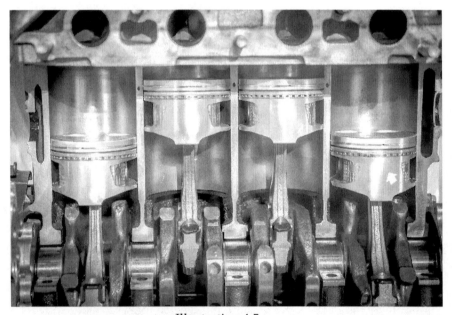

Illustration 4.5

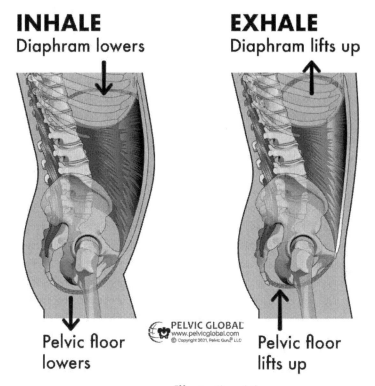

INHALE
Diaphram lowers

EXHALE
Diaphram lifts up

PELVIC GLOBAL
www.pelvicglobal.com
© Copyright 2021, Pelvic Guru® LLC

Pelvic floor
lowers

Pelvic floor
lifts up

Illustration 4.6
Images used with permission from Pelvic Guru®, LLC www.pelvicglobal.com

This "piston movement" should happen if your pelvic floor is working nicely with your breathing muscle (your diaphragm). When you breathe in, your diaphragm lowers a little bit and widens out. Your pelvic floor should do the same—lower a bit and widen slightly. When you breathe out, your diaphragm lifts up and your pelvic floor should also lift up. Yes, your pelvic floor is supposed to contract and lift up slightly when you exhale! That's how the diaphragm and the pelvic floor are designed to work together. And that's why it's crucial to get that system working properly again so you can regain control over your bladder. (Illustration 4.6)

Now, what if the opposite is happening? What if you're thinking, "Hey wait a minute, I thought I was supposed to inhale when I tighten my pelvic floor." Nope, that is not the way your body is designed to work. I'll explain what's really going on when you try to do it that way, and how to fix it if that's the pattern your body is using.

If you inhale when you tighten your pelvic floor muscles, suddenly you have increased the pressure inside your abdominal cavity. And what does that mean for the pelvic floor? More pressure inside the abdomen means more stress and more strain on the pelvic floor muscles every time you breathe. This in turn can increase your chance of leaking urine. Good news, though, this is fixable. You can learn to get your "piston" working well again. It might be easier than you think!

Here's one easy way you can get started on your Pelvic Connection.

I call it **Balls Breathing.**

The name was invented by one of my former clients, the guys think it's genius! It's very simple, really. The only cue you need is this:

"Breathe deep into your balls." *

Simple but effective!

"Balls Breathing" helps your pelvic floor muscles to move correctly with your breathing muscle. It gets that "piston" movement working without you having to overthink it.

Subtlety is the key. Allow the movement to happen, don't try to force it.

To Note: this is just a breathing exercise. I do not expect you to breathe like this 24/7 all the time. This is a "reconnection" activity for your diaphragm and pelvic floor.

This concept is one of the foundations of the Success Plans that we create for our physical therapy clients. Everyone starts with this step. We need to get this Pelvic Connection working before we move on to the next steps of retraining and strengthening.

This is included in the Recovery Toolkit to help you create your own Action Plan.

A Sample Client Success Plan

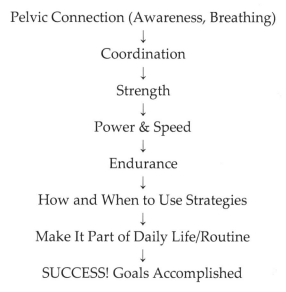

Pelvic Connection (Awareness, Breathing)
↓
Coordination
↓
Strength
↓
Power & Speed
↓
Endurance
↓
How and When to Use Strategies
↓
Make It Part of Daily Life/Routine
↓
SUCCESS! Goals Accomplished

Bladder Basics

What is "Normal?"

As you start your recovery process, you may be wondering exactly where you're headed. Sure, you want to get rid of that annoying and embarrassing leakage. Is there something beyond that?

Many guys bring up the question, "What IS normal bladder function?"

How do you define "normal"?

How should your bladder behave if there was nothing wrong?

Great questions. Let's find your baseline.

If your bladder was in good working order, here's how it should behave:

NORMAL BLADDER FUNCTION BASICS

1. Bladder capacity = 300-400 ml, or about 16 oz. (the size of a Grande Latte)
2. 8 voids per day, 1 or less at night (1-2 voids/night if you're over age 65)
3. Voids are every 3-4 hours
4. Urine stream is strong, continuous, and starts right away
5. Urine is clear or light straw-colored
6. Urine stream should stop completely with no dribbling afterward
7. Voiding is not painful
8. Urge to void sensation is present
9. Able to delay that first urge sensation for at least 15-20 minutes

How does your current bladder function compare? Take the quiz on the next page to find out.

MY BLADDER FUNCTION BASELINE QUIZ

1. Bladder capacity: how much am I voiding when I urinate? (You can measure it or estimate: small, medium, large amount)
2. How many times do I urinate during the day? _____ During the night? _____
3. How long do I go in between voids? _____hours, or _____ minutes
4. How's my urine stream? (circle one answer in a, b, and c)
    a. Strong or weak/slow
    b. Continuous or stop-start
    c. Starts right away or hesitates
5. Does my urine stream stop completely when done? Is there dribbling afterward?
6. Is my urine clear or light straw-colored? Is it dark yellow, brownish, or cloudy? Is it blood-tinged?
7. Do I have pain with urination?
8. Can I feel a sensation of urge to urinate?
9. Can I delay that first urge sensation for at least 15-20 minutes?

Compare your results with the Normal Bladder Function Basics from the previous page. How close is your baseline to normal?
Are you close to baseline? (6 or more questions match with normal)
Are you a bit below baseline? (3-6 questions match with normal)
Are you far below baseline? (0-3 questions match with normal)

This is your starting point, and it can help you with creating your own Action Plan to get your baseline closer to normal. The Recovery Toolkit can provide you a more detailed step-by-step guide.

Keep reading to learn about an important part of the peeing process that you don't want to get wrong!

Peeing Mechanics

No doubt you've thought about the peeing process more than ever before!

How does it really work, and how is your pelvic floor involved?

Your ability to pee properly is controlled by a brain-bladder communication system called Bradley's Loop.[7] See illustration below for a summary of how this works.

When you're ready to urinate, what should happen is this:

- Bladder neck and internal sphincter muscle relax
- Bladder muscle (detrusor) contracts, to squeeze urine out
- Pelvic floor muscles, including external sphincter, relax.

REMEMBER THIS:

When the bladder muscle contracts to let you pee, your pelvic floor muscles should relax!

This is one reason why you should NOT practice Kegel exercises when urinating!

Normal urination is like driving down a super-highway. Your pee starts when you want, flows down the "highway" unobstructed and at a good speed and stops when you want it to. There are several things which can interrupt or alter this pattern of peeing mechanics. These things can act as roadblocks, lane closures, or obstacles:

- Enlarged prostate, which restricts urine flow (like closing down all but one lane of the highway).

---

[7] Claire C. Yang and Gerald W. Timm. "William E. Bradley and his contributions to urology." *The Journal of Urology* 179, no. 5 (2008): 1700-1703.

- Damage to internal urethral sphincter muscle. You've lost one of the main gateways of control.
- Pelvic floor muscles staying tight and constricted during urination. Bradley's Loop can't work like it should. It's like trying to squeeze toothpaste out with the cap still on.

Ever heard of power-peeing? It's when you use more force through the abdomen and pelvic floor to try and push the urine out. A lot of men develop this habit if they've had an enlarged prostate prior to prostatectomy. It's the body's way of compensating to get that urine out. What often happens (and gets overlooked) is that the pelvic floor muscles learn to function incorrectly and develop too much muscle tone. They can actually become tight AND weak.[8]

Now that you have this baseline information, let's move on to learn about the types of incontinence you are dealing with. There may be more than one!

---

[8] Scott, Kelly M. et al. "Individualized pelvic physical therapy for the treatment of post-prostatectomy stress urinary incontinence and pelvic pain." *International Urology and Nephrology* 52 (2020): 655-659.

PISS OFF (Literally)

CHAPTER 5

NOT ALL LEAKAGE IS CREATED EQUAL

Did you know that there are several types of incontinence? Did you also know that you can have more than one kind of incontinence after prostate surgery? Different kinds of incontinence occur for different reasons and may need to be treated in different ways. In this chapter, you will learn about the most common types of incontinence and the reasons why they happen.

TYPES OF INCONTINENCE

Stress Incontinence

Stress incontinence happens when there is stress put on the pelvic floor which is too great for it to withstand. The pelvic floor muscles fail to do their job. When this kind of muscle failure happens, you get leakage. That's what's happening with your pelvic floor muscles when you sneeze, when you lift something, when you sit up in bed. All those activities (even sitting up in bed) put more pressure inside the abdomen. That pressure's got to go somewhere—and often it goes straight down to the pelvic floor. If those pelvic floor muscles aren't strong enough to withstand that stress, if they are not working with the rest of the core muscles, OR if your body is not managing that pressure well, the result is urine leakage.

Urgency Incontinence

Urgency incontinence is when you get that sudden strong urge to urinate. This urge hits you hard and fast and is out of proportion to what you normally feel. You have to rush to the bathroom immediately or you'll start leaking, or worse, have a full-blown accident. One of the main reasons for this isn't muscle weakness. Instead, it can happen when the brain sends signals to the bladder that are way out of proportion—too strong, too loud. Ever seen a 2-year-old throw a temper tantrum? You get the picture then.

Or it's like a microphone that suddenly gets turned up full volume and all you get is feedback. You know how awful that sound is, and all you can think about is TURN DOWN THE VOLUME—NOW!!! That's what's happening with your nervous system in urgency incontinence.

Did You Know... in a normal bladder, when you get that first urge, your bladder is only about half-full? That first urge is like a tap on the shoulder to get your attention, not a megaphone screaming at you and demanding that you go NOW.

Urgency/Frequency
(also called OAB or overactive bladder)

You can have this problem with or without any urine leakage. It can still be quite bothersome. You get that strong sudden urge. You can make it to the bathroom IF you hurry and IF there's a bathroom close by. That urge sensation happens far too often (i.e., frequency). You feel like you're having to pee every 20-30 minutes, but you can't get much out, or you just end up dribbling a lot. This can often happen at night, resulting in you waking up three, four, maybe five times during the night to pee. Now you're frustrated AND losing sleep every night! Your spouse or partner probably isn't too thrilled either.

Urgency/frequency can happen for several reasons:

- overactive nerve signals to the bladder (remember the nervous system drama with urgency incontinence?)
- changes made to the bladder during surgery. As a result, the bladder does not stretch as much and is not able to hold as much volume of urine.
- tension in the pelvic floor or the other soft tissue around the bladder area

Mixed Incontinence

Can you have both stress incontinence and urgency incontinence or OAB? Absolutely, a lot of people do. Sometimes you will have those strong feelings of urgency, but you also leak when you sneeze, cough, or lift. That is often called mixed incontinence in medical jargon.

Now that you know a little bit more about the different types of incontinence, you're going to learn what you can do about it. You will learn techniques and strategies to help overcome stress incontinence (in Chapter 8) as well as the problem of urinary urgency and frequency. You'll be able to take some of those first steps in addressing your problem and stopping those annoying leaks.

We will start with the problem of urgency/frequency. This problem requires some different retraining and strategies to be effective. Continue on to find out how Harold overcame his problem. Although Harold chose a different cancer treatment, this problem can also occur after prostatectomy.

TURN DOWN THE VOLUME (Urgency/Frequency)

Harold's Story

Harold came in for his initial evaluation. He had chosen radiation for his prostate cancer treatment a few years prior. All was going well, but then he began to develop bladder control problems, a common delayed side effect from radiation therapy.

One of his main complaints was the urgency/frequency he was experiencing. He described it as an "on/off switch" that was malfunctioning. The problem? The "on" switch, or his bladder urge sensation, was happening far too often. It wasn't normal and he knew it. It hit hard and it hit fast. The result: he had to stop what he was doing, and hurry to the bathroom, all the while trying to maintain his dignity while inwardly panicking that he may not make it in time.

This happened every 30-45 minutes!

And every time he reached the toilet, trying to pacify his fussy bladder, he was "rewarded" with a weak stream and a wimpy volume of urine that dribbled out. And oh, yes, the post-void dribble at the end.

Harold's "on" switch also got flipped throughout the night. He was getting up four, maybe five times a night, every night. This was driving him—and his wife—crazy!

He wanted to know WHY this was happening and WHAT he could do about it, if anything? The only solution his urologist gave him was medications for overactive bladder. He did not want to go that route. He was starting to dread an upcoming trip to visit his son who lived several states away. If he had to stop to pee every 20 minutes, it would take forever to get there!

What Harold was experiencing is often called urgency incontinence, or urgency/frequency (also called OAB or Overactive Bladder). With urgency/frequency problems, the bladder usually isn't full enough yet or even ready to empty, so you often don't get much coming out. Kind of disappointing after all that nervous system drama!

Harold needed to learn how to calm down his fussy bladder. He was encouraged to know that there were things he could DO himself to make this happen!

So, how can you "turn down the volume" and get a better-behaving bladder?

Below are some simple but effective tips and strategies. Harold learned these during his physical therapy sessions. Which ones will work for you? I don't know.

What I do know is that they will give you more tools that you can add to your recovery toolbox. You can use them anytime, anywhere, when you need them. Simple, very inexpensive (the cost of this book), and no side effects. Can you say that about any OAB medication? I think not!

What to Do for Urgency Incontinence

Strategies for "Holding Back the Tide"

Here are six simple strategies that you can try to "hold back the tide" and get to the bathroom in time. To note: these are all suggestions. Some may work for you better than others. Some may not work at all. Try each one of them for at least one day, one strategy per day. Practice them as needed when that strong urge hits. Pick two or three that work best and use them consistently.

1. **Sit or stand still when the strong urge ("the tide") comes over you.**

I know, this is probably the LAST thing you want to do when that urge hits! But honestly, this is a good immediate way to stop a bladder temper tantrum. Being still tells your brain (which then tells your bladder), to

"SLOW DOWN, you need to take a short time-out, there is enough time to get business done."

2. Diaphragmatic breathing (deep breathing or "balls breathing")

Doing slow deep breathing, from the belly, helps to balance the nervous system, decrease tension in the bladder and pelvic floor, and decrease anxiety levels. It is especially helpful when that urge hits. It's often a good strategy to use to get out of that "fight or flight" mode that you feel when you're rushing to the bathroom!

Be mindful of the movement of your pelvic floor when you inhale and exhale. Increasing awareness of your pelvic floor muscle activity is key in regaining control of your bladder function!

Not sure how to do this breathing? You can refer back to the "Balls Breathing" in Chapter 4.

3. Pelvic floor contractions**

By contracting the pelvic floor muscles, you are helping the bladder muscles to stay relaxed and giving them the signal that it's not time yet.

**Do you know how to do a proper pelvic floor contraction? Chapter 6 will go into greater detail and instruction. By far the best way to learn this is under the guidance of a pelvic floor physical therapist.

***CAUTION: If you also have pelvic pain, your pelvic muscles may be too tight for this technique to work well. You may want to avoid this strategy for now.

4. Distraction

Focus your attention on something else, do an activity that requires concentration (counting backward, writing your "to do" list, etc.).

Have you heard of Square Breathing? It's a particularly effective form of distraction, and a favorite strategy of many of my clients. It combines the elements of distraction with focused breathing, giving you double benefit. Here's how it works:

1. Find a rectangle or square shape in the room—a TV, picture on the wall, calendar, window, etc.
2. Draw an imaginary line around the shape with your fingers. Follow your finger with your eyes. This gives your brain more sensory input for the task.
3. Breathe like this as you follow the shape with your finger. Repeat 3-5 times.

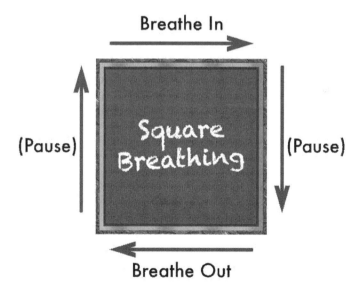

NOTE: "Pause" means you lightly hold your breath as you follow the shape down and back up.

As you get more comfortable with this, you can simply follow the shape with your eyes, using the same breath pattern. Try it—it works amazingly well!

5. Pressure on perineal area

We often do this naturally when the urge hits: squeeze our legs together, cross our legs, or lean forward. What that does is put more pressure on the perineum, the area between the scrotum and the anus. This signals the brain which tells the bladder muscle that it needs to stay relaxed and wait a while longer. Giving you more time to get to the bathroom without rushing.

6. Toe Taps

Sit in a comfortable chair, try to stack your ribcage directly over your pelvis (this helps you sit up straighter). Your thighs should be parallel to the floor. Simply tap your toes up and down for about 30 seconds. Alternate right and left foot. Don't tap both feet at the same time. And keep breathing!

The Easiest Strategy Ever for Nighttime Urgency/Frequency:

You won't believe how incredibly easy this one is—but it really works for most people!

When you wake up at night, ask yourself these two questions:

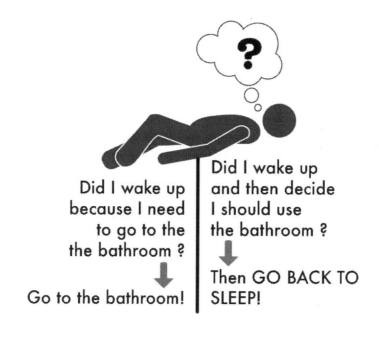

Did I wake up because I need to go to the the bathroom ?

⬇

Go to the bathroom!

Did I wake up and then decide I should use the bathroom ?

⬇

Then GO BACK TO SLEEP!

Seriously, that's it.

Getting up at night to use the bathroom, "just in case," or simply because you're awake, can train your bladder to become overactive. Likewise, staying in bed when you really do not have to urinate can retrain the bladder to return to a more normal voiding frequency.

Can it really be that simple? It was for Harold. Just 2 weeks after trying this, he realized that he really could go back to sleep. His nighttime frequency went down from five times a night to just two times, which is normal for someone his age. Now he (and his wife) are sleeping more peacefully.

How did pelvic floor PT help Harold's urge incontinence and urgency/frequency?

After just 5 sessions and 6 weeks, Harold reported that "the on/off switch seems to be working better." He no longer had to rush to the bathroom, he could take the time he needed and not have an accident on the way. He was able to take long walks again with his wife, something they both were thrilled about. He could "hold back the tide" for a longer time, around 20 minutes. And he was able to urinate with a stronger stream and more volume. "I got my stream back," he proudly announced.

By the way, Harold did make the long drive to visit his son. He had peace of mind and confidence that HE was back in control. His bladder no longer controlled him. He did have to stop along the way but far less often than he originally thought. He enjoyed the journey!

This chapter has focused on managing incontinence caused by urgency and frequency. Before we go over how to deal with stress incontinence, we need to talk about Kegels.

CHAPTER 6

WHAT ABOUT KEGELS?

First things first: let's define what a Kegel is. A Kegel is simply one way to contract your pelvic floor muscles. Chances are you have been told to "do Kegels" following prostatectomy. But do they work? Or rather, do they work as they should, the way they are usually prescribed? The short answer: not usually.

You may be doing Kegels now and they're not working. Or you may be preparing for prostatectomy, TURP or other prostate surgery, and wondering if Kegels are really the magic answer. For many men, they do not deliver the results promised. Here's four reasons why:

Reason #1: Kegels were not designed for men. They were actually made for women. The Kegel, or pelvic floor contraction, was designed by Dr. Arnold Kegel, and he created them in the late 1940's as one part of a much more comprehensive pelvic floor rehab program for women after childbirth.[9] Since they were created for a woman's pelvic floor, they don't do the best job of activating the muscles that a man needs to quickly regain

---

[9] Kegel, Arnold H. "Progressive resistance exercise in the functional restoration of the perineal muscles." *American Journal of Obstetrics and Gynecology* 56, no. 2 (1948): 238-248.

his bladder control. So that might be one reason why Kegels aren't working for you; they may not be targeting the right muscles for your rehab.

Reason #2: Kegels, as they are usually prescribed, are only about strength. But there's a lot more involved than just strengthening the pelvic floor muscles when you're talking about bladder control. After prostatectomy, the prostate is no longer there. In its absence, the pelvic floor now must assume a "new identity" as the main structure to maintain bladder control. You really need to retrain it in a more comprehensive way than just doing Kegels. For example, can you activate your pelvic floor muscles at the right time when doing things like coughing, sneezing, even sitting up in bed? That involves more than strength. Can you coordinate the movements of your breathing muscle (diaphragm), your abdominals, and your pelvic floor when lifting something or exercising? Do you know if the way you breathe is helping your pelvic floor to work well, or making things worse for it?

Just focusing on strengthening—and that's it—might not get you the results that you were hoping for. There's also an important question that is rarely addressed: are your pelvic floor muscles actually too tight? This problem, called pelvic floor hypertonicity, happens more often than you would think. Holding tension, "power peeing," pain, or poor sitting habits can all contribute to this problem. In this case, strengthening could make the problem worse![10]

Reason #3: Kegels are only one tool in your rehab "toolbox." Imagine if you had a big home remodeling project, and all you had in your toolbox was a hammer. How effective would that whole remodeling project be with ONLY a hammer? That's the same way with Kegels. They're designed to really do one thing. One tool in your toolbox of your rehab program. And that's it. You need the right tool to do the job!

---

[10] Scott, Kelly M. et al. "Individualized pelvic physical therapy for the treatment of post-prostatectomy stress urinary incontinence and pelvic pain." *International Urology and Nephrology* 52 (2020): 655-659.

Finally, Reason #4, (and this is what I think is a real disservice to you guys). There's really no training or guidance given on how to do a Kegel. It's not like we were born inherently knowing how to do a Kegel. Most people do not automatically know what that means. Going into the doctor's office and then getting a pamphlet, or maybe a few words amongst a long list of post-op instructions, does not help you learn how to activate those muscles. It does not help retrain the diaphragm, pelvic floor and deep abdominals to work together as a team.[11] It's kind of like learning how to play golf by reading a brochure about it. How effective would that be?

I harp on this because probably 99% of the men who come to my clinic for treatment think they have been doing Kegels correctly (some for over a year), and we find out that they're exercising every single muscle BUT the pelvic floor! Then they have to retrain everything and start back at square one. And that can be pretty frustrating.

So, what do you do now? How do you know if you're even doing your Kegels correctly? What is your next step in getting beyond just Kegels and really getting a handle on this bladder control situation? The next chapters will introduce you to the "Kegels Plus" approach that takes you beyond the basic Kegel to get better results faster.

To go beyond the basic Kegel, you first need to know how to do them correctly. Real time coaching and guidance is best, but if that is not an option, I've written some tips to make sure you're doing your Kegels correctly, and the next chapters will introduce you to the "Kegels Plus" approach to get better results faster.

Let's first review the basic Kegel exercise. I added a few extra tips and instructions that you may not have heard before. Ready?

---

[11] Siegel, A. "The Kegel Renaissance." *Journal of Urology and Research* 3, no. 4 (2016): 1061.

How To Do a Basic Pelvic Floor Contraction, or Kegel

(First step in the "Kegels Plus" approach)

Find where the pelvic floor muscles are. Focus on the front part of the pelvic floor under the scrotum and penis. (Refer back to Chapter 4 for detailed instructions on finding the pelvic floor.)

Tighten/flex this area to contract the muscles. Try one of the following cues to get the right movement:

- Pretend to stop the flow of urine
- "Pull the turtle's head into its shell" (turtle's head = your penis)
- "Nuts to guts" (draw your testicles upward toward your belly)

Here's how to know if you're doing your Kegel correctly:

- You can feel the contraction below base of the penis and scrotum
- Testicles should rise and penis should retract slightly
- Lower abdominal muscles pull in, not bulging out or downward
- Inner thighs, buttocks, and low back muscles are still relaxed
- You are not holding your breath
- Movement of pelvic floor muscles is subtle. You're not doing a max bench press or squat. Don't try to squeeze with all your might.

Are these instructions more helpful than what you've been given?
Ready to upgrade to Kegels Plus? Read On!
This upgraded approach starts with a powerful "secret weapon"...

CHAPTER 7

THE SECRET WEAPON

You already possess a secret weapon to overcome your leakage. It is a powerful tool that you can use, anytime, anywhere. And it's free!

Why secret? My guess is that you've never been told about it. You've never been taught how to use it strategically. How to use it to fight your leakage problem—and win!

I'm talking about breathing.
YES. BREATHING.

Can it really be that simple? For many guys, yes it can be.

The piston analogy from Chapter 4 explained how the diaphragm (your large breathing muscle) and the pelvic floor muscles work together. It's a normal movement pattern—or at least it should be. Can you take advantage of this, and use your breathing to help get your pelvic floor working better? In the simple words of one client, "Absolutely yes."

How can you learn to use your breath to slow down or stop urine leakage? Here are a few tips to get you started. These work well for most guys in general. It works especially well if you have stress incontinence.

What to Do for Stress Incontinence

Strategies for Controlling the Floodgates

1. Stop Holding Your Breath

Are you a breath-holder?

Think about it. When you do things like getting out of bed, lifting something, etc., do you tend to hold your breath?

Why is that a big deal? In these situations, holding your breath can increase the pressure inside your abdomen. It may not feel like much to you, but it may be too much for your pelvic floor to handle, especially after surgery. The result? Leakage.

So, what to do? How can you get out of that breath-holding habit? The first step is becoming aware of it. Once you're aware of it and when it's happening, you can work to DO something about it and make changes. The next step is learning to Exhale with Exertion.

2. Exhale With the Exertion

When you exhale, the diaphragm contracts and lifts up. The pelvic floor should follow suit and also contract/lift up. An exhale also activates the deeper abdominal muscles, which work in tandem with the pelvic floor.

Exhaling acts as a natural pressure valve for your abdomen! (Which is why holding your breath can be problematic.)

Another bonus, if your pelvic floor and diaphragm are working together, every time you exhale you are exercising your pelvic floor muscles!

You may be wondering; how do I know if my pelvic floor really is working with my diaphragm? Am I doing the correct movement when I exhale? Here is a simple self-assessment to find out:

Fold a washcloth or small towel into a square and sit on it (this should help you feel your pelvic floor movement more easily.)

Try one or more of the following activities. Pay attention to what your pelvic floor is doing:

- pretend you're blowing out a candle from far away (use a slow, long breath)
- fake a cough
- say "HA HA HA" loudly (be prepared to start laughing!)
- try to blow up a small balloon

Which direction does your pelvic floor move? Up, away from the washcloth? Or downward into the washcloth? If you feel it moving up, away from the washcloth, the movement pattern is correct. If you felt it pushing down, or you don't know, the diaphragm and pelvic floor muscles may not be working together as a team. You may need to do some basic retraining first to get your system moving properly.

Now that you understand this movement pattern better, you can try using it during three basic everyday activities: getting out of bed, lifting an object, and standing up from a chair.

Getting Out of Bed

First, avoid sitting straight up in bed. (Photo 7.1)

That puts too much pressure on your abdominals, pelvic floor, and bladder, and greatly increases your chances of leaking.

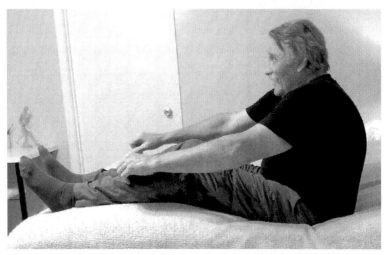

Photo 7.1, Photo Credits Carol Barr, Jason Barr

Try this instead: (Photos 7.2, 7.3)

Sitting up in bed: Roll to one side first. Then, EXHALE as you come up to a sitting position.

Lying down onto bed: Lie on your side first. EXHALE as you bring your legs up onto the bed. EXHALE as you roll over onto your back or your other side.

Using your breath strategically can help to stop those leaks when sitting up in bed or when lying down in bed!

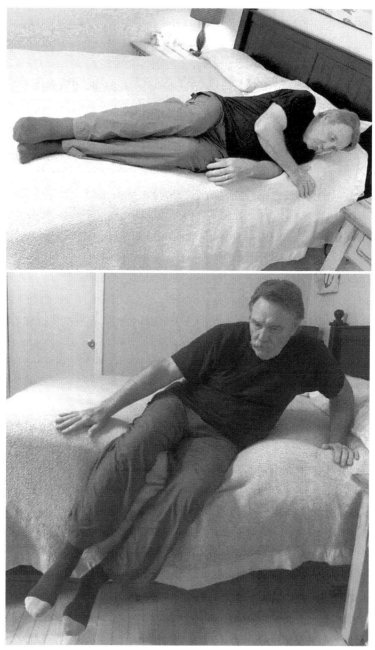

Photos 7.2 and 7.3, Photo Credits Carol Barr, Jason Barr

Lifting an Object

Whether it's a bag of groceries, golf clubs, or weights at the gym, how you breathe when lifting is so important.

Do NOT lift like this! This position puts too much strain on your back and on your pelvic floor. Holding your breath when you lift doesn't help.

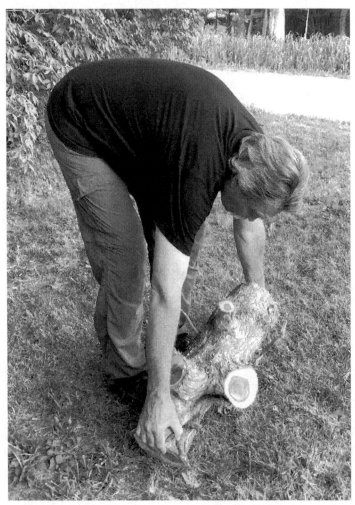

Photo 7.4, Photo Credits Carol Barr, Jason Barr

Instead, do this: Use good body mechanics, and breathe!

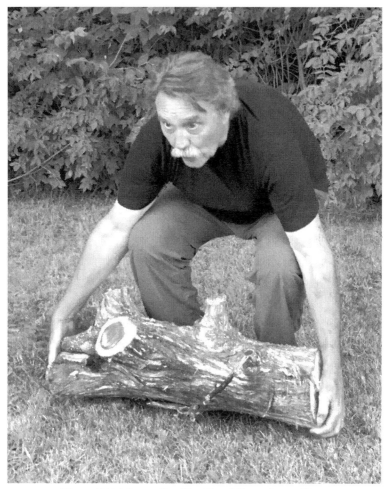

Photo 7.5, Photo Credits Carol Barr, Jason Barr

EXHALE right before you start the lift and as you come up to standing. This helps with the pressure management in the abdomen as you are lifting the weight and makes it easier for the pelvic floor to handle the extra load.

Standing Up From a Chair:
EXHALE as you stand up. That's it.

Do a self-check: Did you leak when you stood up or sat up in bed? If so, was your pelvic floor lifting up or pushing down when you exhaled? Is there some retraining that needs to be done?

Did you leak a little less, or not at all? You're on the right track, keep practicing.

The result: Many men find that when they add the breathing component, they can do these activities with less leakage, or no leakage at all.

3. Get Expert Help When Needed

In some cases, the exhale may not be enough to change the leaking. There may be more going on that needs to be addressed or you may need some one-on-one guidance to get those muscles working as a team.

Introducing the "Kegels Plus" Approach

Getting control over your incontinence involves pelvic floor and core retraining. That involves movement patterns. And that involves the entire body. Another reason why Kegels alone don't work for most men.

The Difference

What makes the "Kegels Plus" approach different from traditional Kegels or strengthening?

It's a Whole-Body Approach.

You know quite well that prostate cancer treatment affects more than just your prostate. We need to get your whole body involved with your recovery, not just a part of your pelvic floor.

It Involves Coordination/Teamwork.

For the best results, you need to train the pelvic floor to work with the diaphragm, with breathing, and with the abdominal muscles. These are not separate elements. They're designed to work together as a team.

It Involves Pressure Management.

Your body may need to un-learn some old habits and learn some new ones to keep that pressure low inside the abdomen.

It Involves Purpose

For these new movement patterns to stick, they must have purpose. They need to become part of your everyday routine. Being associated with a functional task helps them become better integrated into your brain and more likely that you'll continue with them long-term.

With "Kegels Plus," you can retrain your pelvic floor muscles with purpose: while you get ready in the morning, drive your car, do those home repairs, or work out at the gym.

Jack was unaware of this concept of movement with purpose. He had been doing his Kegels faithfully as his doctor suggested, while lying down—for a year. Kudos to him for being so consistent! However, he still had some incontinence. He couldn't figure it out. He had gotten steady improvement, but after about 6 months, his progress stopped. Despite his efforts he never got beyond that, and he was frustrated.

This could be one reason why. Jack was only given ONE exercise, in ONE position. One movement in isolation. If Jack had learned how to use this exercise in a functional way—in a way that had purpose (a way that his brain saw as purposeful), would he have continued to improve? I think so.

The 3 Steps of the Kegels Plus Approach

You'll be seeing this Kegels Plus approach throughout the rest of the book. These three steps will become a common theme for you, and you can apply them to your own recovery journey.

Step #1: Pay attention to your pelvic floor.

Step #2: Get your pelvic floor moving with the rest of your body. Teamwork is key!

Step #3: Have a plan, a strategy, a system in place.
Apply what you've learned and find a way to keep going. Stay the course for long term success.

How the Kegels Plus Approach Works: Vincent's Story

"This is such a sensitive problem for me. Am I ever going to be free from this?"

Vincent came to my clinic at the suggestion of his urologist. It was about two months after his prostate surgery. He was given the typical post-op handout for Kegel exercises and practiced them faithfully every day. No change. He was not seeing any results.

Vincent's problem sounded like activity-specific incontinence. I asked him to tell me what specifically seemed to bring on the leakage. He was especially bothered by two things:

1) Getting Up Out of a Chair

Vincent stated that he would lose urine nearly every time he stood up from a chair. He was very embarrassed by this. He was afraid that he would leak through his Depends briefs, or that others around him would notice the smell of urine. Vincent even had stopped wearing shorts because of this, a particularly bothersome thing as it was the middle of summer.

2) Getting In and Out of Bed

Bedtime was the worst. Every time Vincent sat up in bed or lifted up his legs to get into bed, he leaked urine. Sometimes it was so bad that his pajamas and the mattress got wet. This was very distressing for him. He couldn't stand it!

During his initial evaluation, the first thing I asked him was, "Can you show me how you're doing your Kegel exercises?" "Of course," he said. He got up onto the treatment table (leaking in the process) and lay down on his back. (To note: he was only doing Kegels in one position, lying down).

He then performed a series of squeeze-clench-tilt-thrust-arch movements that worked every muscle in his abdomen, hips and thighs; everything EXCEPT the pelvic floor! Here's what I saw:
- Butt clenching
- Abdomen bulging out
- Pelvis strongly tucking in
- Inner thighs squeezing together
- Low back arching then flattening
- Little to no activity in pelvic floor or perineal area

(By the way, he complained of low back pain after doing his Kegels! Can you see why?)

"Well?" he asked, hoping I would praise his excellent technique. When I told him what I observed, he stared at me, astonished and a little deflated.

"You mean I've been doing these wrong this entire time?"

"No worries, Vincent. What's important now is that you're here. And you can and will learn to do these differently." So, we got to work. With some guided instruction, basic muscle retraining, and unlearning some bad habits, by the end of that first session Vincent was able to do the exercise correctly. He felt more encouraged.

Not so fast... Vincent went to sit up on the table, and his smile immediately turned into a frown. "I leaked again," he told me. "I don't understand. I'm doing the Kegels correctly now. Why didn't it work?"

Secret of the Breath

I asked Vincent this question: "Did you hold your breath?"
"What do you mean?" he replied.
"Do you tend to hold your breath when you do this (sit up in bed)?"
He paused for a moment, then answered, "I really don't know. "I've never thought about it."
"Well, then, let's start thinking about it," I encouraged.

Vincent began learning Step 1 of the Kegels Plus approach. He paid attention to his breath (or lack thereof) during these movements of getting on and off the table. It's the same kind of movement he does when he gets in and out of bed. Sure enough, he discovered that he WAS holding his breath every time.

As I often tell my clients, becoming aware of a problem is the first step in overcoming it.

Why is holding your breath such a big deal? And how could this affect your leakage?

It's a simple matter of pressure management. You read about this earlier in Chapter 4. When you hold your breath during a movement (sitting up in bed, even rolling over in bed), there's more pressure built up in the abdominal cavity. More pressure is placed on the pelvic floor muscles as well. Even more pressure if you sit straight up in bed, as Vincent did! Your pelvic floor muscles may not yet be strong enough or be able to react quickly enough to counter this pressure increase. The result: urine leakage.

Let's throw a little physics into this scenario: lever arm length. This factor was important for Vincent. He is a tall man with long legs. Think about it from a physics point of view:

Long Legs = Longer Lever Arm

Longer Lever Arm = More Force created at the fulcrum (i.e., the abdominal and pelvis areas)

More Force through Abdomen + Underactive or Weak Pelvic Floor Muscles = Leakage

Given this scenario, what physics changes could Vincent make to reduce his chances of leakage?

Change #1: Shorten the lever arm.

Change #2: Reduce the amount of force.

Change #3: Change the condition of the pelvic floor muscles.

Read on to find out how he made these changes.

Kegels Plus step #1: pay attention to your pelvic floor
He became aware of the specific things that made him leak:
- Holding his breath when:
    - Sitting up in bed
    - Getting out of a chair
    - Lifting his legs to get into bed
- Sitting straight up in bed
- Lifting his legs up and arching his back when trying to lie down

Kegels Plus step #2: get your pelvic floor moving with the rest of your body
He learned simple ways to change positions or movement patterns to reduce the pressure and strain on his pelvic floor muscles:
- Rolling or turning onto his side, bending his knees, then using his arms to push himself up to a sitting position (physics changes #1 and #2)
- Lifting up his legs with knees bent, after he turned onto his side (physics change #1)
- EXhaling with the EXertion (physics changes #2 and #3) when he did these position changes:
    - Side-lying to sitting
    - Sitting to standing
    - Back-lying to side-lying
- Changing seat angles
    - Vincent had trouble with leakage when getting out of his car or getting off the couch. When I observed him doing this, I noticed that his knees were higher than his hips and buttocks. There were two problems with this position:
        - His pelvic floor muscles were lengthened and had to contract more forcefully,
        - More force was required for him to stand up.

THE SECRET WEAPON

o   The solution: adjusting his car seat or raising the height of the couch so that his knees were not higher than his hips. Less force required to stand up = less force placed on pelvic floor (physics changes #1 and #3)

Kegels Plus step #3: have a plan, a strategy, a system in place

Vincent was amazed at how quickly he saw results. Within one week, he was able to get into bed and get out of bed without leaking!

The problem was consistency. Vincent did not yet have a Plan (the third part of the Kegels Plus approach), so his movements were not yet second nature. As time went on, he and his wife came up with some strategies that worked very well for him.

Now, Vincent is able to stay dry when getting in and out of bed and has the confidence in knowing that he has mastered this skill. Now it's second nature, "I don't have to even think about it anymore."

It's amazing how much difference a few simple movement changes can make. Another reason why we need to go beyond just doing Kegels to get results that last.

UPGRADING TO KEGELS PLUS:

Go to the "Kegels Done Right" instructions at the end of Chapter 6. Add the breathing and the abdominals into the equation for a more coordinated "teamwork" effort. (Illustration 7.1)

Here's how to sequence your breathing with a pelvic floor contraction:

—**INHALE** when you **RELAX** your pelvic floor muscles

—**EXHALE when you TIGHTEN**/flex your pelvic floor muscles (you should not inhale when you tighten)

—**Lower abdominals** (below the belt) **should pull IN when you tighten**/flex pelvic floor muscles, not bulge outward or downward

INHALE
Diaphram lowers

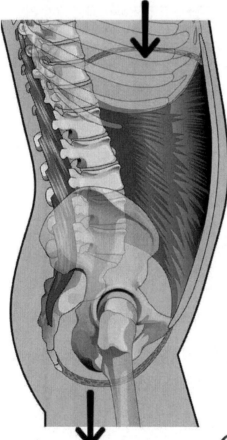

Abdominal wall expands

Pelvic floor lowers

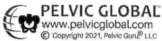

PELVIC GLOBAL
www.pelvicglobal.com
© Copyright 2021, Pelvic Guru® LLC

Images used with permission from Pelvic Guru®, LLC www.pelvicglobal.com

EXHALE
Diaphram lifts up

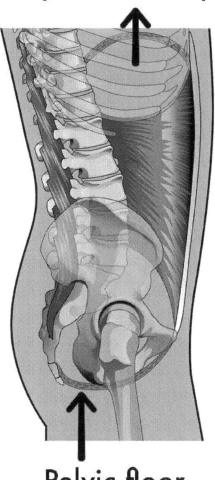

Abdominal
wall
contracts

Pelvic floor
lifts up

Images used with permission from Pelvic Guru®, LLC www.pelvicglobal.com

HOW to self-assess: (no biofeedback machine needed)

- Place your fingers lightly on the skin between your scrotum and rectum. You should feel that area tense and lift up slightly when the muscles contract. You'll feel the area let go and come down into your fingers when the muscles relax.
- Look, use a mirror. If you're doing it correctly, the penis should lift up slightly and maybe retract a bit. You should also see the scrotum lift up slightly.
- Sit in a chair or on an exercise ball. You'll feel your pelvic floor lift up very slightly when you contract and return to the chair/ball surface when you relax.

CHAPTER 8

GETTING BACK TO LIVING LIFE!

"Now that we're keeping you alive, how do you want to live?"
—*Dr. Rachel Rubin, M.D.*

Getting your urinary control back and enjoying life again involves more than just doing Kegels. In this chapter you will learn some helpful tips and suggestions on how to get back to:
- exercise
- work
- social outings
- travel
- life without diapers or pads

Back To Exercise

Joe was a very active guy in excellent physical condition. He could run circles around men half his age! He ran, did intensive workouts at the gym, and was training for an upcoming mountain-climbing excursion. This got interrupted by the unexpected discovery of prostate cancer. With the expert guidance of his doctor, he chose the option of radical prostatectomy.

Although Joe was told he would probably be fine after the surgery, he still had the resulting incontinence. This bothered him greatly. He was not expecting to have to wear the continence briefs. He rejected the advice to wait 6-8 weeks to see how much of his bladder control returned on its own. "No way I'm doing that," he said. "I don't want to just wait around; I need to stay active!" Joe decided to take a more proactive approach and began physical therapy as soon as he could. He began preparing his body BEFORE his surgery (we call that "prehab")!

As a physical therapist, I am a big advocate for movement-based therapy. Our bodies are designed to move, and they crave movement. Movement is an important part of the healing process.

Many of my clients have been encouraged to do this by their medical team. Diet and exercise are being recommended more often now as part of the overall recovery process. I think that's great! However, most men are still given very little guidance on how to make that happen. That big gap still exists. This section is written to help give you something beyond generic advice of "go exercise." You'll learn how exercise can help your recovery, some general guidelines for exercise after prostate surgery, and tips on how to get started or restarted.

Benefits of Exercise[12,13]

Exercise can do amazing things, including:

- Reduces depression
- Improves fatigue
- Boosts mood
- Improves cardiovascular health
- Improves strength and endurance
- Improves sexual health
- Improves quality of life
- And...improves bladder control

The first tip I'll give is: Start early!

If you're reading this because you have a family history of prostate cancer and want to be proactive in your health, start NOW.

If you've gotten a troubling report on your PSA or prostate exam but no active cancer yet, start now!

If you've already had your surgery and have clearance from your doctor, start now!

Let's discuss the first steps in getting started.

General Exercise Guidelines

Go Slow—Ease back into it

Don't go from "Restricted" (0-6 weeks—lift 10 pounds or less) to "Everything" (6 weeks—do whatever).

Joe found this out the hard way. He was doing great on the Stairmaster at the gym, felt very confident and decided to increase his steps from 400 to 1,000 the next day. The result? Incontinence got worse! He backed off the

---

[12] https://www.pcf.org/news/prostate-cancer-loves-couch-potatoes/

[13] https://zerocancer.org/learn/current-patients/maintain-qol/exercise-and-activity

steps to 400 again, and the problem self-resolved. He learned that 1,000 steps were above his tolerance level at that time; he needed to ramp up his activity more gradually. When he did that, his leakage remained manageable.

How might this work for you? For example, if you want to get back to running, start first with a light stroll. Progress to a brisk walk → light jog → running on level surfaces → running on inclines and uneven surfaces.

Some basic self-progression guidance: take note of how much your leakage amount changes when you increase your activity level. Are you able to maintain status quo when going from brisk walk to light jogging? Great, continue with the jogging. Or, did you find that your leakage got a lot worse? Then back off the intensity or the duration of the jogging. Still leaking a lot? Your tolerance level might not be ready to move to jogging; go back to the brisk walking for a while. Your pelvic floor muscles need time to gain sufficient strength and endurance to do their job (i.e., keep you dry) during your exercise.

Breathe!

Avoid breath-holding during exercise. It does not help you lift better, walk faster, or improve your coordination. The one thing it does contribute to is more urinary leakage! That is because of the poor abdominal pressure management with breath-holding. You can refer to Chapter 4 for a refresher on this important concept.

More is not always better!

It's okay to work the muscles to fatigue, but not beyond that. A tired muscle is not going to perform better. It will just encourage other muscles to compensate for the problem. That doesn't fix your main problem. It just sets the stage for other problems.

No good will come out of trying to force more work out of an already-fatigued muscle.

I always tell my clients that I'd rather have them do five reps correctly than push through ten or more with poor form and using the wrong muscles just to finish the reps. Classic example: the guy who does 100 Kegels straight out of the gate because he thinks that will strengthen his pelvic floor faster (when in reality his pelvic floor can only handle three to five reps). He ends up exercising every muscle BUT the pelvic floor, and he wonders why he is still leaking.

No "No Pain No Gain"

This is not a good rule to follow. You may experience some discomfort and soreness as you get back to exercise, that's normal. But to push beyond pain, especially after prostate cancer surgery or treatment, is not recommended. It doesn't gain you anything.

Listen To Your Body.

What does that mean exactly and how do you do it?

Basically, it means pay attention to what you're doing, and be aware of the warning signs:

- Do you catch yourself holding your breath?
- Do you find yourself straining and tightening up during a stretch or movement?
- Are you feeling tightness or discomfort creeping up that doesn't go away?
- Do you notice that you're starting to substitute other muscles or sacrifice good form just "to get the job done"?
- Are you having pain anywhere, especially "down there"?
- Do you just have a sense that your body is not up to the task that day? Might want to heed that!

Be Aware of Pelvic Floor and Sphincter Fatigue

This usually occurs later in the day and is one reason why you may continue to leak more towards afternoon or evening. One reason it's happening is that your pelvic floor muscles haven't yet gotten the endurance, the "staying power" that they need to maintain bladder control throughout the entire day. This will improve as you continue to work on your pelvic floor strength over time.

One suggestion for now is to change the times that you exercise. Try a walk in the morning. Try working out earlier in the day rather than after work.

Another option is to modify the activity itself:

- Instead of playing 18 holes of golf, play 9 holes
- Instead of 1 set, start with just 1 game
- Instead of running that 5K, try walking it
- Instead of cycling uphill, cycle on level surfaces

Lighten Up on The Squeeze!

Don't try to clench or squeeze your pelvic floor all the time. You'll just tire the muscles out and probably worsen the leakage.

Don't try to squeeze to the max either—lighten up a bit. The pelvic floor doesn't always need to contract to its fullest extent for every movement.

Be Prepared

Do wear a pad or even a brief if needed while exercising if you notice increased leakage. Have an extra one handy "Just In Case."

By the way, Joe did succeed in achieving his exercise goals. He followed all of the tips that you just read about. After three and a half months post-surgery, he was able to resume his cardio and strength training level with 90% less leakage. He also did his mountain-climbing excursion and was happy to report to me afterward that he was now "98% dry." No more diapers, no more pads. An occasional drip here and there but it didn't bother him anymore. Most importantly, he regained his confidence and self-esteem. Did the prehab make a difference? We think so. The latest research supports this.

Exercise Suggestions, Specific Activities*

*Note: these are only suggestions and not a prescription or exercise program. I'd highly recommend reaching out to a qualified exercise or fitness professional for individual guidance and training. Please refer to Chapter 11 for these resources.

Walking

It seems so simple, but you can turn walking into a fitness activity!

Numerous studies have already proven the benefits of walking as a form of exercise. For you as a prostate cancer patient/survivor, walking as exercise can help reduce stress, strengthen your muscles, lower your risk of cardiovascular disease, maintain bone health, boost your immunity, and improve your quality of life.

Walking at a brisk pace is a great example of Movement with Purpose. Here's a few tips to get the most benefit out of this activity: (Photo 8.1)

1. Be mindful of your posture
   a. Back is relaxed and upright
   b. You are not leaning forward or stiffly arching backward.
2. Let your arms swing gently and freely.
   a. Avoid holding them stiffly by your side.
   b. Fun fact: did you know that your natural arm swing helps to keep rotation movement in your mid-back, which in turn can help your pelvic floor muscles work better?
3. Keep your abdominal muscles gently engaged and working.
   a. Belly is not pooching out
   b. Stomach is not sucked in tightly

4. Watch where you're going
    a. Be aware of possible obstacles in your way, but don't constantly look down at your feet.
    b. (If you have balance issues or are afraid of falling, please consult a physical therapist or other exercise professional to address this.)
5. Pick up those feet!
    a. Let your feet clear the walking surface.
    b. Walk "heel-toe," which means starting a step with your heel, and ending it by pushing off with your toes.
    c. Try to avoid shuffling your feet or walking flat-footed. This can make a big difference in your balance and in your hip, leg, and pelvic floor strength!
6. Wear shoes with good arch supports and cushioning, if possible. This will act as a shock absorber for both your feet and your pelvic floor muscles.

You can walk anywhere! If you're not able to get outside, you can simply walk around your house or apartment. That will work just fine. Other options are an indoor mall, community center, your office building, or your local shopping store.

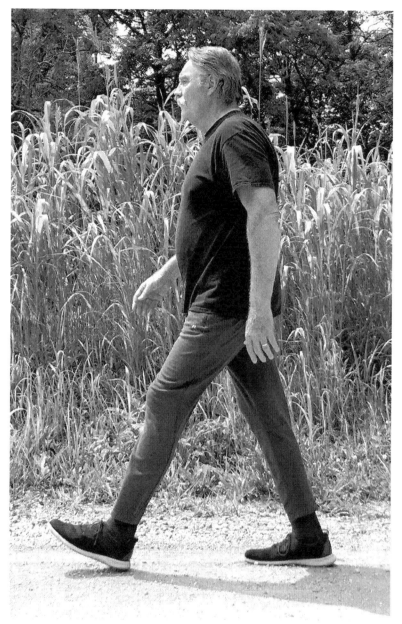

Photo 8.1, Photo Credits Carol Barr, Jason Barr

Yoga

Yes, real men do yoga! The ancient practice of yoga was originally for men only. It's much more than stretching or flexibility.[14] Yoga teaches breath control and connection of the breath to the pelvic floor, which you already know is crucial to recovery. Yoga is a great way to gain muscle strength, reduce stress, and work on that "listening to your body" awareness. It's also a fantastic way to get your pelvic floor muscles in good working order, since it promotes both strength and mobility. You need both for good continence control.

Unfortunately, there are very few men's yoga classes or online programs out there. If you're a beginner to yoga, I'd suggest starting with a gentle restorative class if it's available. An aggressive "yoga burn" class isn't going to get your bladder control back faster. Stick to the basics. It's best to have a yoga instructor who actively teaches modifications and monitors your movements throughout the class.

Tai Chi

Have you heard of Tai Chi? This movement practice is known to enhance body awareness and balance. Its slow controlled movements are more gentle but very purposeful and can be a good physical challenge. It also emphasizes breath control. Tai Chi can provide a different but effective way to regain pelvic floor strength and control.[15]

---

[14] Kaushik, Dharam et al. "Effects of yoga in men with prostate cancer on quality of life and immune response: a pilot randomized controlled trial." *Prostate Cancer and Prostatic Diseases* 25, no. 3 (2022): 531-538.

[15] McGee, Robert W. "Tai Chi, Qigong and the Treatment of Cancer." *Biomedical Journal of Scientific & Technical Research* 34, no. 5 (2021): 27173-27182.

Resistance and Strength Training

There are many proven benefits to strength training in general. The research specific to post-prostatectomy is not as robust.[16] However, the clinical findings are very strong (pun intended).

How should you begin strength training? If you've never done it before, the best suggestion is to seek out a qualified personal trainer who has experience with cancer rehab, or a physical therapist. They can guide you in how to progress safely with your training.

If you are already familiar with resistance training, here's a few tips:

- Again, avoid holding your breath when you lift.
- EXhale during the EXertion part of the lift. Remember to coordinate that exhale with a pelvic floor contraction for the best results and reduced or no leakage!
- Start out slowly, gradually increasing the weight amount.
- It's also helpful to strengthen the large muscles that attach to the pelvis: your quadriceps (front of thigh), adductors (inner thigh), abductors (outer hip) and hamstrings (back of thigh).
- You can still achieve strengthening through bodyweight exercises; no weights or dumbbells are necessary.

Sports are a great way to stay active, but several of them do tend to increase the risk of leakage. These include:

- Golf
- Pickleball
- Tennis
- Basketball
- Running

I'm not saying to avoid these forever, but to be aware and prepare.

---

[16] Lopez, Pedro et al. "Resistance exercise dosage in men with prostate cancer: systematic review, meta-analysis, and meta-regression." *Medicine and Science in Sports and Exercise* 53, no. 3 (2021): 459.

Back to Work

"I'm kind of nervous about going back to the office. What if I pee all over myself during a meeting?"
—Rick, age 59

You may plan to return to work after your initial recovery time. Working from home can make this transition easier. However, not everyone is able to work from home. Going back to the office or working from multiple locations can present different challenges and worries. Some common concerns:

- Increased overall stress level. At first, your stress level may be higher as you and your bladder deal with an environment different than home.
- Less control over your schedule compared to your recovery time.
- Less control over when and where you take bathroom breaks!
- More interruptions that may occur in an office environment.
- Worries about being around coworkers (will they ask me about my problem? Can they smell my urine leakage? Can I make a quick exit to the toilet without drawing attention?)
- Not knowing where the bathrooms are when traveling to different locations.
- Figuring out how to change continence briefs or pads in a public restroom.

Here are a few tips for making that transition back to work a little more comfortable and a lot more successful:

Bring a "Work Survival Kit" with you.

This could include extra pads, individually-packaged wipes, fabric spray, change of underwear, etc. Place items in a non-clear plastic, cloth, or paper bag. It's easier and more discreet to bring into the bathroom stall with you.

"Double Up" if needed.

If you still need to wear full continence briefs and are concerned about overflow leakage, stick a pad or shield inside your brief. That offers you a double layer of protection. You can do the same "double up" with a pad plus a guard or shield.

Discreet pad disposal.

How to dispose of your wet pads or briefs in a public men's restroom without drawing attention? Place them in a small dark-colored plastic bag and drop into the trash. Another option is to use a "gender-neutral" or "unisex" toilet room if available. Such toilet rooms are often private, larger in size, and contain a disposal bin for pads.

Do "body checks" throughout the day.

Do you notice any muscle clenching patterns? Are you holding your breath? Does your pelvic floor feels tense and stressed out? Take a few seconds to change that using the strategies you're learning in this book. A few deep breaths ("balls breathing") can help right away. Then get back to your work.

Take short movement breaks more frequently, at least once every hour. Your pelvic floor needs the exercise.

Does your work involve sitting? Do several pelvic floor contractions before getting up. EXHALE when standing up from your chair.

Do 3-5 pelvic floor contractions in the bathroom stall AFTER urinating. Not only does that help strengthen your pelvic floor, it can also help to reduce that post-void dribble. For a refresher on how to do a proper Kegel, read the end of Chapter 6.

Ease up on the coffee at work, at least during those first few weeks. Caffeine is a common bladder irritant which can increase your urinary urgency and frequency. Too much of it during this transition could create problems for your bladder.

Skip the lunchtime martinis and soft drinks for now. Like caffeine, alcohol and carbonation could result in a more temperamental bladder than you'd care to deal with at work.

Feeling overwhelmed by that list? The good news is, this is temporary!

As you regain bladder control, you will need less padding and less protection from leaks. You will need fewer bathroom breaks. You will be able to enjoy coffee break again. You will also learn how to fit your "Kegels Plus" pelvic floor retraining into your work routine. Chapter 9 will help you create your own long term Action Plan.

Back to Social Drinking

"Laura, don't tell me to give up my wine."

"When I'm out with the guys, I want to still have a beer with them. Do I have to give that up forever?"

Rest assured; I won't tell you to give up alcohol forever after your prostate surgery. Do check with your surgeon, however, for any medical reasons why you should not be drinking. Whether it's one drink or five, consuming alcohol will likely pose a challenge for your bladder. Why? Alcohol nearly doubles your urine production. It also relaxes your muscles (including your pelvic floor muscles).

Beer has the greatest effect, followed by wine and then hard liquor. Why is that? Think about the difference in volume: 12 or 16 oz of beer vs. 5 or 9 oz of wine. You'll drink more volume of beer than you would wine or hard liquor.

A few tips if you'd like to go out with the guys and have a drink or two:

1. Moderation! Control how much you consume.
2. Don't chug! Drink more slowly to avoid a big rush of urine production.
3. Wear a pad or shield just in case or have one in your pocket.
4. Drink sitting down vs standing. Before standing up, give that pelvic floor a few quick contractions to minimize or eliminate leakage with this position change. (And remember to EXhale.)
5. Wear dark-colored pants or shorts if you're worried about leakage.

Back to Travel

Incontinence is not a problem that affects only the person who has it. Sometimes it can have a ripple effect, impacting the lives of entire families. This is Jerome's story.

Jerome was a physical therapist but had no training in men's health issues. His father had a TURP procedure to fix some non-cancer prostate issues, and afterward had to deal with—you guessed it—urinary incontinence. Jerome's father hadn't been referred to physical therapy for his recovery, nor had he expected this to be such a problem. Jerome himself felt very ill-equipped to advise his father on what to do. This bothersome side effect had caught both of them off-guard, and they were understandably frustrated.

His father's incontinence was more than bothersome. It disrupted their entire plans as a family. Before the procedure, Jerome's parents had made plans to travel from Florida to Massachusetts for a family wedding. Now those plans were on hold and might be canceled altogether. The realities of travel were rather harsh:

- How many Depends briefs or pads will I have to pack?
- If flying, will there be a bathroom nearby when I need it?
- What if I can't get to the bathroom in time on the plane?
- Will others on the plane be able to smell my leakage?
- If driving, how many bathroom stops will I have to make? It will take forever to get there.
- What if I wet the bed in the hotel?
- How many times will I have to excuse myself during the wedding or reception to change my briefs or pads or to change my pants if the leakage is really bad?
- Will I really be able to enjoy myself knowing that I'm leaking every time I stand up?

These questions and concerns finally won out, and Jerome's father canceled their visit.

Jerome was really disappointed by this. This was the first time that their entire family would have been together in over five years. They were all looking forward to seeing each other, laughing, having a great time, and catching up in person. And now, because of this one problem that wasn't getting addressed, they would be missing two very precious members of their family at this event.

Can you relate? Have you had to cancel travel plans or change them because of your incontinence problem?

Here are a few helpful travel tips that you can try out on your next journey, whether driving or flying. These are some things that you can do to keep your bladder happy and healthy, to "hold back the tide" and make it a little bit further along your way, and to make the trip more pleasant.

Travel Tip #1: Stay Well Hydrated

I know you're tempted to drink less because you don't want to go to the bathroom a lot. However, that irritates your bladder even more because it concentrates your urine. Your bladder does not like urine concentrate!

Besides, dehydrating yourself is just not a good thing to do to your body. Your cells need that water to function well. I don't want you to end up with other problems because of dehydration. If you don't like plain water, add a little bit of natural flavoring. You can purchase water enhancer flavorings, or you can make your own. Avoid those that contain sugar or artificial sweeteners. Carbonated water may not be your best choice right now, as carbonation is a common bladder irritant.

Travel Tip #2: Holding Back the Tide

You're driving down the road and you suddenly get that urge that you gotta go—NOW! But you don't see any rest stops close by. You might be able to stop at the side of the road, but sometimes even that is not an option. What to do?

It's important to know that the first urge you get usually means that your bladder is only half full. In most cases, if you ignore it or concentrate on something else, that first urge will go away. This allows the bladder to fill up more and then send the second urge signal that says, "It's really time to go now!"

If ignoring the first urge doesn't work for you, you can do some "balls breathing" and/or a few pelvic floor contractions. This may hold back the tide until you can stop. Contracting your pelvic floor muscles helps the brain to tell the bladder to relax because it's not quite time to go (refer back to Bradley's Loop in Chapter 4). This gives you more time to get to a stop with control and dignity.

Travel Tip #3: Be Still. And Breathe!

When you finally pull into that truck stop, you may be tempted to rush out of your car to get to the bathroom as fast as you can. That kicks your body into "fight or flight" mode and ramps up your nervous system (including the nerves going to the bladder). The result? Your bladder gets ramped up, too, giving you signals of urgency that are too strong and happen too fast.

How can you counteract this? **Be still.** This may sound like the exact opposite of what you want to do! But I encourage you to try it! When you park, take a few seconds to sit still. Take a deep breath or two. Then calmly get out of your car. Stand still. Take a deep breath and then walk (not run) to where the bathroom is. I'm sure the last thing you want to think about is taking your time, but it really does help your bladder control.

Travel Tip #4: Avoid Common Bladder Irritants

You have just stopped at a gas station or a restaurant. You need a drink and a snack. What should you choose to keep your bladder behaving at its best? Avoid the oversized soft drinks that are full of sugar, caffeine, and carbonation. That's three major bladder irritants all in one drink! (Do you really NEED 24 ounces of soda??)

If you need that cup of coffee to stay alert while driving, go ahead. Keep it small (I recommend 12 ounces or less) and go easy on the added sugar or creamer.

Gas station snacks are convenient but may contain hidden bladder irritants. Sugar and artificial sweeteners can create a cranky bladder for some. Spicy foods can also bother your bladder. One ingredient that you may not know about is monosodium glutamate, or MSG. This can also be a bladder irritant, especially for urinary urgency/frequency. It is often an ingredient in processed or packaged foods—yep, including convenience store snacks! Check the label first and see if monosodium glutamate is listed as an ingredient. Then you can decide if you really want that snack item.

Travel Tip #5: Bring a "Travel Survival Kit"

Several prostate cancer survivors have created their own version of this: a small, neutral-colored bag where you can place pads or briefs, small plastic bags for wet disposals (try colored or white small wastebasket bags that aren't see-through), and individual packets of wipes. I use Dude Wipes* in my clinic, but you can find a variety of options at stores or online. This kit should be easy to carry, lightweight, and free you from unwanted attention. One of my former clients wears cargo pants or shorts that have ample-sized pockets for his items.

Travel Tip #6: Bring Extras, Plan for "Just In Case"

It's obvious but bears repeating: if you don't want to find a store to buy briefs or pads during your travels, bring enough along! Consider what kind is most absorbent. It may be worth paying a little extra for a brand like Tena* to have the extra absorbency during your travels.

There is such a thing as men's "pee proof" underwear. It doesn't stop leakage, but it does a pretty good job of containing mild leakage. That way you can avoid having to change pads or briefs while traveling and keep your trousers dry.

Wearing boxer brief underwear will help to better contain any leakage and will help to keep pads or shields in place.

Dark shorts or pants will help hide any unexpected accidents.

Happy Travels!

*Dude Wipes and Tena are some of the brand names that I often recommend. I'm not making any money by promoting them or any other product, I just think that they work well and are of good value.

Back to Wearing NO Diapers or Pads

Jo Milios Pad Weaning Protocol

Finally, I will end this chapter with Getting Back to Wearing NO Diapers or Pads! Joanne Milios, an Australian physiotherapist and top expert in prostate cancer rehabilitation, has created a protocol for men to reduce their dependence on Depends*.

Quite often we find that men are wearing briefs and pads longer than they really need to. Going through this protocol can help with bladder retraining and reduce the need for continence products. Give it a try. What have you got to lose, except for a drawer full of Depends?

Before we begin, let's define some terms. Shopping for these continence products can be a daunting task. There's different names, different thicknesses and sizes. How do you sort that out to find what you need? Do you know what a brief is, what the words "pad," "guard," and "shield" mean? A lot of guys don't know. Heck, I didn't really know until I started writing this book!

In this case, I think that a picture is better than a lot of words. (Photo 8.2) Each product is labeled based on the Pad Graduation Process on the following pages. You may find that these terms vary among product companies.

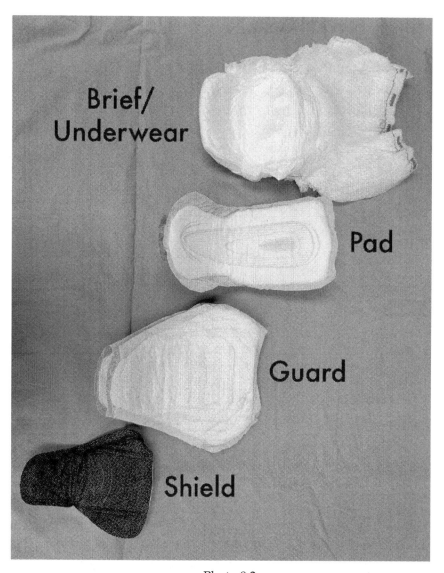

Photo 8.2

"Ditching The Depends": A Pad Graduation Process, based on Dr. Joanne Milios' Pad Weaning Protocol

[Dr. Jo Milios (PhD) MACP B.Sci (Physiotherapy) Western Australia]

1. Wearing full briefs day + night
2. Graduate to wearing maximum strength pads day + night
3. Not much leakage at night? Graduate to wearing a shield at night
4. Shields dry for three nights in a row? Ditch them! You don't need them anymore at night. Sleep in underwear without shields
5. Wait to apply pad in the morning: instead of immediately putting on pad, wait 5 minutes. Increase wait time 5 minutes a day. This helps your body and bladder get used to not wearing a pad all the time.
6. Continue to wear a pad, with less thickness, during the day. Change to thicker pad when going out of the house or when doing more strenuous activity.
7. Reduce to minimal thickness pad during the day. Continue with only underwear at night if you are still leak-free when you're sleeping.
8. Remove pad before bedtime, gradually increasing the time between pad removal and bedtime (start with 5 minutes before bedtime, increase time by about 5 minutes per day). This allows your bladder to get used to more time spent in the evening without a pad.
9. Reduce to a guard or shield for daytime use. Continue to increase time in the morning and in the evening without the guard.
10. Reduce to wearing NO pad during the day. (You will get there!) Place a small shield in your pocket "just in case" for reassurance.
11. When you forget that the shield is in your pocket, you are DRY.

(To note: for a while you may want to have a backup pad or shield handy when drinking alcohol or when doing very strenuous activity)

Congratulations, you have graduated from Depends*!
Enjoy your new-found freedom and control.

*Depends is a brand name for continence briefs and pads. There are many other brands available to choose from.

PISS OFF (Literally)

CHAPTER 9

STAYING THE COURSE

"Do I need to do these exercises the rest of my life?"

That's one question I often get from clients. Sometimes it's a clarifying question. Sometimes it's a concern. I think that underneath this question are other ones, often unspoken:

- What if I fail myself?
- Will I always have to work at this? (Like a task that can never be finished.)
- What if I stop? Will I ruin everything?
- How do I stay consistent?
- I don't trust myself to stay accountable

It's a valid concern. Short answer: yes, you will have to keep doing the exercises and activities you've learned. You know that they work for you.

Since your prostate is no longer there, your body relies even more on the pelvic floor muscles to keep you dry and prevent leaks. The pelvic floor muscles are skeletal muscles, just like your biceps, and like any other skeletal muscle, they need to be exercised to stay in good working order.

In other words: "USE IT OR LOSE IT"

You may often hear it this way at your urologist follow-up appointments:

"You'll have to do these exercises (Kegels) for the rest of your life."

To me, that sounds self-defeating right from the start. It's not very motivating or encouraging. It seems impossible.

I challenge you to look at it a different way:

"Make this (Kegels Plus approach) part of your daily routine."

Now THAT you could do. It sounds possible, even probable, for a couple of reasons:

First, as you now know, regaining your bladder control involves more than just doing a few exercises. It's more than strengthening. It's retraining your body (and brain) to work in a way that gives your pelvic floor muscles the best shot at working well.

Second, it's quite simple to add this into your daily activities. James Clear, author of the best-selling book <u>Atomic Habits</u>, talks about this concept. One term he uses is "habit stacking." It's basically stacking a new activity onto an already established habitual one. Find several things that you do every day, which are already habits. Add one pelvic floor retraining activity into this habit. Use these established habits as prompts, to remind yourself to do your exercise/activity at the same time.

Here are some examples from actual clients:

- Practice your "balls breathing" when you are waiting at a stoplight
- Do 10 reps of pelvic floor contractions while:
  - you're waiting for food to reheat in the microwave
  - you turn on the water for your shower
  - you're waiting in line for anything
- Add breathing into your daily meditation practice

- Do a quick pelvic floor contraction (coordinated with exhale) every time you:
  - get up out of a chair
  - sit up in bed
  - get out of your car
  - cough or sneeze
  - lift golf clubs or groceries from your car trunk
- Do 3-5 quick pelvic floor contractions after every void/urination
- Make the Kegels Plus approach part of your workout routine

It's really quite simple to do. As you can see, there's so many ways to habit-stack. You can keep up with your Kegels Plus approach while you go about your daily life. And it doesn't have to take any extra time!

Simple, yes. Not always easy. It's challenging to develop and maintain a new good habit. Many of us fall off the wagon after a while. It doesn't mean you're lazy, have no willpower, or are a failure. It's just human nature.

The trick is to find those positive triggers, those prompts that can help you stay consistent. That's why habit-stacking works so well. You may be thinking, that's great and all, but I still need some kind of reminder to DO the exercise and keep at it. Your wife or partner nagging you about it every day may not be the best prompt!

Here's some helpful suggestions for possible reminders:

- phone alarm
- reminder alerts on phone or computer calendar
- write it in your daily To Do list
- bright sticky notes strategically placed where you'll see them:
  - on the microwave door
  - below the TV
  - across from where you usually sit

- o on the wall or cabinet behind the toilet; in good view when you stand to urinate
- o on the sunshield of your car

Try several and see which works best for you.

It can also be very helpful to get accountability from someone else. Find an accountability buddy. Enlist the help of a friend or another prostate cancer survivor. This could be in-person or virtual. Sometimes we need another person to make sure we do what we said we would. Like I've said, no man is an island. No man should have to walk the journey of prostate cancer treatment—or rehab—alone! Besides, having a buddy around can make this more fun.

CHAPTER 10

PROVE IT!   LATEST RESEARCH

It can be discouraging to read about research for men's health issues. There's not a lot available, and study results can vary or be less than impressive. Why is that? One reason is that the human body is incredibly and wonderfully complex. Prostate cancer is complex. No two cases are identical, no two tumors are exactly alike. There are many variables that are out of our control. However, some of the latest research shows surprising and promising results. Let's look at a couple of those studies:

Pelvic floor muscle training in radical prostatectomy: a randomized controlled trial of the impacts on pelvic floor muscle function and urinary incontinence[17]
2019, BMC Urology
Joanne Milios, Timothy Ackland, Daniel Green

---

[17] Milios, Joanne E., Timothy R. Ackland, and Daniel J. Green. "Pelvic floor muscle training in radical prostatectomy: a randomized controlled trial of the impacts on pelvic floor muscle function and urinary incontinence." *BMC Urology* 19, no. 1 (2019): 1-10.

This one is truly groundbreaking! It's quite recent, well done, and showed very positive results.

What makes this one so unique?

1. It started with PREHAB—Pelvic Floor Muscle Retraining BEFORE surgery (preparation)
2. It targeted different pelvic floor muscles than previous studies
3. It took into account the difference between fast-twitch and slow-twitch fibers (Chapter 4)
4. The pelvic floor muscle training was done in standing position, vs. lying down

All of these points are very relevant to men. This is a study designed specifically for the MALE pelvic floor, not a male version of a female pelvic floor study. **It's the first of its kind.**

The study was divided into two groups and into two different time frames: BEFORE and AFTER Surgery.

BEFORE Surgery:
Each group was given a different therapy program:

GROUP A: Got the "usual care," starting 5 weeks before surgery:
- Bladder retraining education
- Two sessions of standard Pelvic Floor Muscle training, which works more of the posterior (back) pelvic floor muscles. Training was done in three positions: lying down, sitting, and standing.

GROUP B: Given "high intensity" program, also 5 weeks before surgery:
- Bladder retraining education

- Two sessions of higher intensity Pelvic Floor Muscle training exercises
- Exercises targeted both the slow-twitch (endurance) muscle fibers and the fast twitch (power and speed) muscle fibers of the pelvic floor.
- Exercises were done in standing position only
- Specific cues were given ("stop the flow of urine") to ensure a correct and complete contract/relax movement.
- Correct technique was verified by Real-Time Ultrasound. This gave a much more objective measure of muscle movement.

AFTER Surgery:

Therapy continued for both groups after removal of the catheter. Each group received a specific exercise program for 12 more weeks.

GROUP A: Continued with the same exercises as they had done pre-operatively. Exercises were done in the same postures as before: lying down, sitting, and then standing.

GROUP B: Exercises continued and included both fast-twitch and slow-twitch muscle training. Intensity was higher than Group A. Exercises were done in standing position only.

After 12 weeks post-surgery, the results showed that:

74% of GROUP B men (high-intensity training) was dry, compared to 43% in GROUP A

DRY = NO MORE LEAKAGE. FULL CONTROL BACK.

Even at 2 weeks post-surgery, 14% of men in GROUP B were dry, vs 4% in GROUP A!

Other improvements noted in GROUP B:

- Faster return of bladder control
- Faster speed of pelvic floor muscle contractions
- Longer hold times of pelvic floor muscle contractions = better endurance
- Better quality of life

One thing that is so different about this study is that it started 5 weeks before surgery and continued after surgery for another 12 weeks.

This is very promising! Of course, this is only one study. The body of research on prostate cancer rehabilitation is still small. More studies are needed.

If you're interested in reading the entire study, it is publicly available.[18]

This study makes sense from both an anatomical and a functional perspective.

- It was designed for men. It was not a male version of a pelvic floor study for women.
- It targeted the muscles—and more specifically, the muscle fiber types—that a man needs in order to have bladder control and maintain continence.
- The pelvic floor training exercises were done in the functional position that made the most sense: standing. Most men experience urine leakage when they are standing, or when going from sitting to a standing position.

---

[18] Milios, Joanne E., Timothy R. Ackland, and Daniel J. Green. "Pelvic floor muscle training in radical prostatectomy: a randomized controlled trial of the impacts on pelvic floor muscle function and urinary incontinence." *BMC Urology* 19, no. 1 (2019): 1-10.

- It adds the crucial "prehab" phase! This sets you up for even better success and quicker recovery.

Kegel Exercises After Prostate Surgery Called into Question[19]
Jan 15, 2020, Renal and Urology News
John Shieszer

Is It Really All About Strength?

Another recent study challenges the current protocol of giving Kegel exercises to everyone following prostatectomy. The title could be misleading, so I encourage you to look beyond that and read the entire article.

Many physicians, and even physical therapists, assume that all you need to do after your surgery is strengthen your pelvic floor muscles and you'll be fine. This study asks the question, "what if weakness isn't the main problem? What if the pelvic floor muscles are also too tight?"

Weak AND tight? Yes, that is possible! It happens more often than you might think. Go back to Chapter 6 for a refresher on how this can happen.

Typically, all the focus is on strengthening, with the assumption being that the pelvic floor muscles are weak. Has anyone even checked your pelvic floor to confirm that it's just weakness?

This study challenges the medical community to look beyond just strength or weakness, to address and treat pelvic floor muscle tone more accurately and appropriately. And THAT is our specialty as pelvic health physical therapists!

---

[19] Schieszer, John. "Kegel Exercises After Prostate Surgery Called Into Question." Renal & Urology News. January 15, 2020. https://www.renalandurologynews.com/home/news/urology/prostate-cancer/kegel-exercises-after-prostate-surgery-called-into-question/.

The study found:

- The majority of the men had overactive pelvic floor muscles, not just weakness, contributing to their incontinence and pain. (overactive = muscles are working too much, have too much tone)
- Men often develop pelvic floor overactivity after surgery, and any type of pelvic floor dysfunction can lead to incontinence.

It is one of the first studies to show that pelvic physical therapy can be helpful to ease PAIN after prostatectomy.

Again… Not just weakness. Not just about strength.

As mentioned before, you need to address the pain and muscle tightness as well as the muscle weakness.

There were some limitations to this study. Although it had some important findings, it wasn't designed to find out if pelvic floor exercises would be helpful to patients after surgery.

One thing I don't like about this study is the long wait time participants had after their surgery—SIX MONTHS! Why must men "wait and see" for up to six months before they are referred to pelvic rehab? My thoughts on this: if they had gotten physical therapy sooner, maybe they wouldn't have developed the muscle overactivity and the resulting pain. What do you think?

Case Study: Gary

Success Story, Based on the Latest Research

"Gary" was referred to me for physical therapy three months following his radical prostatectomy. He was still having severe incontinence which basically kept him home bound. He was going through 10 briefs per day. He was unable to work, he could not even get out of a chair without full urine loss. He was very frustrated. "I hate wearing these stupid Depends!" he told me.

Gary had tried Kegels the best he could. Nobody had really shown him how to do them correctly. He was an active man in his late 50s. He certainly did not want to spend 6-12 months to "wait and see" if his bladder control returned. He wanted to DO something about it himself! So, he began to seek out other options. He heard about pelvic floor physical therapy and asked if he could be referred to a therapist for treatment. That's how we met.

At Gary's first appointment, we addressed the first problem: lack of information and guidance. He learned exactly what the pelvic floor was, how it worked in relation to the prostate, and why it is important for bladder control and sexual function. Just having that information provided him with reassurance and some hope.

Gary quickly learned that his problem was not just pelvic floor weakness. He did not know how to use these muscles to stop urine leakage. You've already learned that after the prostate is removed, the male pelvic floor must assume a "new identity" as the main component for bladder control. To do that, it must be strong but also know how to work with the rest of the body as a team.

And so his rehab journey began. Gary had to relearn how to use his pelvic floor muscles. He had tried to learn Kegels, but they didn't help. We found out why when he came to see me: he was exercising every muscle BUT the pelvic floor! His upper abdominals, glutes, hamstrings, and inner thigh muscles were getting a workout, but the pelvic floor muscles were barely moving.

Backed Up by Research

Just as medical research has advanced early detection and treatment methods for prostate cancer, physical therapy research has led to improvements in therapy interventions. That leads to better results. We used methods based on the latest research studies, including the Milios 2019 study, to create Gary's treatment plan. Gary's research-based treatment included:

Exercising in the Standing Position

We began exercising standing up as soon as possible. In Gary's case that was easy; he was physically ready and had been doing Kegels lying down for far too long.

Activating the Right Muscles

We emphasized activating the **front part** of the pelvic floor, not just the back part (Kegels focus on the back part). How did he learn that? It starts with proper verbal cueing. We tried different verbal cues and found the best ones to get his "front passage" muscles firing.

The cue that was used in the study was: *"Pretend that you're stopping your urine stream."* We also tried different cues that had worked well for other guys: *"Pull the turtle's head back into its shell"* and *"Nuts to guts."* I know, it sounds silly. But it really works! These cues specifically target the front part of the pelvic floor, which includes the muscles around the urethra and at the base of the scrotum and penis.

"Biofeedback" done differently

Biofeedback was another research-based intervention we used. The original study used Real-Time Ultrasound (RTUS) to verify correct muscle movement. Consider it the ultimate in biofeedback! As we did not have access to this technology, we used readily available items to help the body "find" the pelvic floor muscles: a tall mirror for visual feedback, fingertips or folded washcloths for touch feedback when standing or sitting. Once Gary could find the right muscles, he could start retraining them.

Higher Intensity

Higher-intensity levels of exercise got faster results in both strength and endurance of pelvic floor muscles. We looked at the standard retraining protocols (like Group A was given) and doubled the number of repetitions and sets. Gary did both slow contractions (for endurance and strength) and quick contractions (for power and speed). He was given speed and time challenges each session, which he liked. This was a very different approach than the standard advice of "do at least 100 Kegels a day."

We also worked on other things to address Gary's specific needs:

Reducing pelvic floor muscle tightness

Yes, tightness! Many men develop increased tightness in their inner thighs, hamstrings, and pelvic floor after surgery, often a result of guarding and trying to "hold it in," or from doing Kegels incorrectly. A tight pelvic floor cannot contract or move like it should. Gary had very tight hamstrings and inner thigh muscles, probably from trying to hold his urine in. This tightness also needed to be addressed.[20]

Breathing and Coordination

---

[20] Scott, Kelly M. et al. "Individualized pelvic physical therapy for the treatment of post-prostatectomy stress urinary incontinence and pelvic pain." *International Urology and Nephrology* 52 (2020): 655-659.

Coordinating the breath with pelvic floor movements is a key part of successful rehab. The diaphragm muscle and the pelvic floor muscles are designed to work together, like a piston. Incorrect breathing, or worse, breath-holding, makes it harder for the pelvic floor to work correctly to stop urine leakage. Gary made a startling discovery: his breathing habits were actually part of the problem. Once Gary stopped holding his breath and used his breathing strategically, his pelvic floor muscles contracted 50% more in just a few minutes!

Making it Functional

Learning to use the pelvic floor muscles correctly when doing daily activities, especially activities which provoke leakage. In Gary's case, the biggest offenders were sitting up in bed, getting out of a chair, and putting on those dreaded Depends. Gary learned that with a few simple changes in his movement and breathing patterns, he could immediately reduce the amount of leakage during those activities. After just two weeks, he was able to sit up in bed with no leakage at all!

Transitioning Back to Life

Learning how to self-assess, self-progress with returning to exercise, and how to start weaning off those Depends briefs. Gary was particularly excited about that.[21]

Results!

After just 6 sessions in 10 weeks, Gary was down to only two pads a day. He had returned to working full-time, riding his motorcycle, and even traveling by plane. His incontinence didn't get in his way anymore. Even if his progress had ended there, he was happy with the results he'd achieved. "This is manageable now, it's no longer overwhelming me," he said. (I expect Gary to make a full recovery, however.)

---

[21] Dr. Joanne Milios' Pad Weaning Protocol. Dr. Jo Milios (PhD) MACP B.Sci (Physiotherapy) Western Australia.

I often wonder, if Gary had started physical therapy earlier, even **before** his surgery, could he have gotten results faster? I think so. Remember the results from the 2019 Milios study that we followed—74% of the men were dry 12 weeks post-prostatectomy. DRY. That means no pads, no nothing. Full bladder control restored.

Will everyone who follows this kind of treatment plan get these results? Probably not. There are a lot of factors that can determine the results you may get. Gary was a great candidate for pelvic physical therapy and had several things in his favor. His surgery was straightforward with no complications and no resulting muscle injury. He was fairly young, physically active, and had no problems with incontinence or erectile dysfunction prior to his surgery. Your results may vary depending on your age, physical condition, and extent of your surgery. The good news is, even if you don't feel you are an "ideal candidate," you still can do something to improve your condition.

Gary was also willing and able to put in the time and effort needed to get his bladder control back. In my experience, those who commit the time to learn and practice the exercises usually do quite well, even with other medical complications.

The results from the Milios study are truly remarkable. They are very promising for advancing the quality of care that our survivors could receive. Gary certainly benefited from it. This is not yet the standard of care in our country; my hope is that it will be, and soon. Our guys deserve it.

I asked Gary at his last appointment what advice he would give other men about pelvic floor rehabilitation after surgery. Without hesitating, he replied: *"Start Early."*

PISS OFF (Literally)

CHAPTER 11

RESOURCES FOR MEN

Phil was mindlessly scrolling Facebook one evening, unaware that a solution was around the corner.

He had been dealing with significant urinary leakage for over five years following his prostatectomy. Like many men, he was told that he shouldn't expect to be incontinent after his surgery, that most men don't have that problem after the surgery. Phil was never given the option of physical therapy to retrain his bladder or his pelvic floor. After one year, he was still leaking like a sieve. He had the male bladder sling surgery to fix this. It did nothing. He was still leaking.

His last resort, so he was told, was a different surgery procedure. He did not like this option. Phil was a very athletic man, a competitive cyclist, and he hated not having any control over this. Even though the success rate of this second surgery is high, it was not what he wanted to do.

So, Phil took it upon himself to find a different answer. One day, he was browsing Facebook when he came across an ad for pelvic floor physical therapy. He stopped scrolling and read further: it said that pelvic physical therapy could help men who had bladder problems after prostatectomy.

"Hey, THAT'S what I need!" he exclaimed.

He took action and responded to the ad. That's how I first met Phil. It was my ad. Phil called me directly to find out more. Could this really work for his problem? Could this really help even after 5 years of incontinence?

Phil decided that he had nothing to lose by trying this. He learned the "Kegels Plus" approach that you have already read about. This was new information to him. He did not achieve 100% cure, but he was able to reduce his leakage to the point where he just needed one pad during his cycling competitions. That was much better than urine freely running down his leg by the time he reached the finish line! Phil was very satisfied with the results he got and saw no need to proceed with the second surgery. He had achieved his goals.

It would be great if all men were given this option by their surgeon, beforehand or afterward. The reality is that doesn't happen very often. It's not yet the standard of care. Prehab is not even thought of, and rehab after surgery is still rarely considered. This leaves many men—perhaps even you—trying to figure it out on their own.

Scouring the Internet or YouTube for help can be frustrating. There's really not much out there. It can leave you with more questions than answers: how do I know if I'm doing this right? Is this source legit? Do these people really know what they're talking about?

That's why I included this chapter. I've heard from so many guys how difficult the process is to find help for their incontinence. Not to just manage the symptoms—there's always Depends, pads, or medication for that. But to actually DO something about the problem themselves.

I've gathered some of the latest and greatest resources to help you through that process. It's not an exhaustive list, it will continue to change, and I've probably left some things out. But I hope that you find it to be a good start, the next step in regaining control over your bladder so that it no longer controls you!

Directories—Find a Pelvic Health Professional Near You

If you'd like one-on-one guidance and treatment, there are several national online directories that can help you find a qualified provider who specializes in men's health issues. Such providers would include physical therapists, occupational therapists, exercise and fitness specialists, physicians, and sex therapists.

Two online directories that I highly recommend are:

Pelvic Global   https://pelvicguru.com
Pelvicrehab.com   https://pelvicrehab.com

Self-Advocacy

As you read in Phil's story, sometimes you are not given these options, yet you know there must be a better way. How do you advocate for yourself? How do you bring up the topic with your surgeon or urologist in a way that's a respectful win-win for you both?

Often just mentioning these options is enough to start a healthy dialogue. Your doctor usually wants you to have better outcomes! He or she may be thrilled to learn about other options out there that worked for you, are proven to be effective, and could help other patients.

If the conversation doesn't go so well and your medical provider is opposed to considering any other options, giving you no reason why, perhaps a second opinion would be in order.

Another part of self-advocacy is becoming an active learner. Educate yourself about your prostate cancer care journey, your treatment options, and what you can do about possible side effects. Many of my clients agree that knowledge is power. It puts you in a better position to actively participate in your own healthcare and advocate if needed for the kind of care you want.

Where do you start? It can seem quite daunting to begin your own research. A few pointers to help with the process.

- Look for a source that continues to update information. Prostate cancer information is changing rapidly with many new advances and developments. You'd be surprised how many websites, even from cancer centers, are not updated. Find something that is staying current with the changes.
- Be wary of sources that make outrageous claims or promise 100% cure IF you buy their stuff, etc. If something looks too good to be true, it probably is not true.
- Stories or blogs from other prostate cancer survivors can be very encouraging and motivating. They are sharing with you what they have learned. Keep in mind that what worked for them may or may not work for you. Their stories can, however, help you to move forward in your journey.

Would you like a few suggestions to get started? Here are some sources that I use for my professional education and that I recommend to my clients. Not all are local or U.S.-based. I like a global perspective!

Continence Foundation of Australia:
https://www.continence.org.au/who-it-affects/men/prostate

Prostate Cancer Foundation of Australia:
https://www.prostate.org.au/media/468680/understanding-urinary-problems.pdf

Prostate Cancer UK:
https://prostatecanceruk.org/prostate-information/treatments/surgery
https://prostatecanceruk.org/prostate-information/living-with-prostate-cancer/urinary-problems

Prostate Cancer Foundation, U.S.:
https://www.pcf.org/about-prostate-cancer/prostate-cancer-side-effects/urinary-dysfunction/

Zero Prostate Cancer, U.S.
https://zerocancer.org

"The Penis Project" Podcast
https://thepenisproject.org/
Available on Spotify. This podcast shares the stories of everyday men dealing with prostate cancer or who have had prostatectomy. Hosted by Jo Milios, Australian pelvic floor physiotherapist, and Melissa Hadley Barrett, nurse practitioner and sexologist. Highly recommend this one!

Survivor Support Groups

Is there a local prostate cancer survivor support group in your area? Drop in to one of their meetings, meet other survivors and listen to their stories. Such groups can often be a much-needed resource and offer practical help as well as mental and emotional support as you walk this journey. You won't be alone.

If you don't feel comfortable going to a group meeting, or if you live in a rural area, you might want to check out online groups or forums. It may be a good way to get connected with other survivors.

Below are a few suggestions to begin your search for a group that can help you walk this journey and not be alone. You can find a local group, an online group or forum, a private Facebook group, even support for spouses and caregivers.

Prostate Cancer Foundation Support Group Guide (wide variety of private Facebook groups)
https://www.pcf.org/patient-resources/patient-navigation/support-groups/

Zero Cancer Support Group Guide (in-person and virtual online groups)

https://zerocancer.org/get-support/black-mens-prostate-cancer-initiative

https://zerocancer.org/get-support/peer-support/find-a-support-group/

You can also call your local hospital's cancer center to find out what support groups they offer.

Did you also know... "The Penis Project" Podcast can be a virtual support group for you, since many of their episodes are about prostate cancer?

CHAPTER 12

NOT THE END...

George called my office one day. He was in a hurry to schedule an appointment with us.

"I don't have much time to work with you, Laura; here's why..." He was going to be moving overseas in less than 2 months. An unexpected diagnosis of prostate cancer threatened to cancel that move. He decided that he was not going to let this ruin his plans. George took swift action and had a radical prostatectomy. He was well-informed of the possible side effects. His second action step was to start pelvic floor physical therapy immediately.

We got to work. We had 35 days.

Was his goal to be 100% dry in 35 days? No. (Although he wished that would happen!)

Was my expectation that he would be 100% leak-free by then, problem solved? No.

What WERE his expectations and what were mine? What would a successful outcome look like for him? Together, we agreed on this:

- He would have a timetable of changes to expect during his recovery.
- He would have the tools and strategies to manage things on his own after he leaves.

- He would have the confidence level to use these strategies to get the long-term results that he wants.

Time was against him, but George did have the advantage of in-person physical therapy sessions. He got a personalized plan for his specific needs. He was able to talk through and process some of the worries and concerns he had about now being a man without a prostate. You can't get that personal touch from a book (including this one).

However, he was able to achieve many other benefits that **you** can also accomplish through this book:

- Knowledge of your man parts, where they are, how they should work, and why this Kegels Plus approach can help with incontinence.
- Having an Action Plan to solve this problem.
- Knowing what to expect and setting reasonable expectations and goals.
- Knowing that there is something you can DO, yourself, to help your situation.
- Knowing how to track your progress (instead of just guessing).
- Being validated—that this problem IS important, that it DOES matter, and that you are NOT alone!
- Learning strategies for long-term success that work! (Instead of just "doing exercises the rest of your life.")
- HOPE!
  - That you CAN do something.
  - That things CAN get better.
- Results!
  - No more leaking, OR if some leakage remains, you can handle it.
  - You control your bladder; it no longer controls you.

When George moved overseas one month later, he was not 100% cured. He still had to wear pads at times. He still worried about how his bladder would behave during travel and in a new environment. He still had uncertainties. But...

He was 100% more equipped and empowered. His leakage had reduced to a level which he felt was manageable. He had knowledge that he didn't have before. He learned skills and strategies which he could use any time and in any setting.

He still had worry and anxiety about the final outcome, but he had an inner reassurance that he would be okay. He knew what he needed to do—and to continue doing—to get the results he wanted.

Above all...he now looked forward to enjoying this next chapter of life. He wasn't afraid that his leakage would ruin everything. He had what he needed to navigate the rest of the way. And if he needed additional help or guidance, he knew where to find it.

This is what I hope for you as well. That you can use this book to find hope, to find strength, and to find a plan that helps you get back to living life and enjoying it, without forever depending on diapers or pads.

No man should have to walk this journey alone. If you found this book helpful, I'd ask you to please share the information with someone else who needs it. Share it with your urologist or oncologist! Help us to spread HELP and HOPE.

As my late friend Caesar Blevins would say: "Teamwork Makes the Dream Work."

You don't have to just "live with it"!

PISS OFF (Literally)

RECOVERY TOOLKIT

Build Your Own Action Plan

I wanted to include this Recovery Toolkit to assist you in creating a personalized plan of action. Consider it a toolbox that you will be filling with many different "tools" you can use to solve your leakage problem. These tools will be in the form of checklists, tips, strategies, and plan-building guides. You've already seen several references to this Toolkit in the previous chapters. The Recovery Toolkit can be used as a companion to the book or as a stand-alone feature.

Each "tool" is listed in alphabetical order, not in order of importance. This will give you a general understanding or a brief reminder of what each tool is. It will also help you to know which tools are best for your situation. The Progress Notes section following will help you learn HOW to use these tools in an easy to follow, step-by-step format.

For best results, I would advise beginning with the big picture—create your overall Action Plan first. Below is a guide to help you find what you need to build an Action Plan that works for you.

What You'll Need to Build Your Action Plan:

BUILDING YOUR ACTION PLAN

GOALS — What results do you want? Write them down here.

Be as specific as possible. Go beyond "I want to stop leaking." Some examples include: sleep through the night and wake up dry, go out with my spouse/partner without wearing diapers, play 18 holes of golf without leaking, return to my regular workouts at the gym, etc.

STEPS — How will you get there? What steps will you take? Refer to Sample Action Plan and Progress Notes.

TIMELINE — How long might this take? Write down a date. I would suggest at least 12 weeks as a reasonable goal, based on my clinical experience and the latest research.

Here is the sample client Success Plan that you saw in Chapter 4. Use this as a guide to build your own Action Plan.

If you prefer to write out a more detailed Action Plan, you can use the blank NOTES pages at the end of this Recovery Toolkit.

Now you will have more tools than just Kegels to work with!

MY ACTION PLAN (Sample)

Pelvic Connection (Awareness, Breathing)
↓
Coordination
↓
Strength
↓
Power & Speed
↓
Endurance
↓
How and When to Use Strategies
↓
Make It Part of Daily Life/Routine
↓
SUCCESS! Goals Accomplished

What are my goals?

How long should this take?

YOUR RECOVERY TOOLKIT TOOLS LIST

Pre-Surgery Questions Checklist
(Not a complete list. Feel free to add your own questions.)

What do you need to know before your surgery?
- What kind of surgery will be done? (robotic, trans perineal, etc)
- Will nerve-sparing procedures be done if possible?
- How long will I be in the hospital?
- When can I expect to get the catheter out?
- What should I bring with me to the hospital? (clothing, continence pads or briefs, etc.)
- If I live alone, do I need to have someone stay with me? For how long?
- When can I start driving again?
- Will I have any lifting or exercise restrictions?
- How long do I need to be off work?
- When can I start to return to exercise?
- What are the warning signs of problems that need immediate medical attention?

What problems might you have after surgery?
- Incontinence?
- Erectile dysfunction?
- Pain?
- Changes in penis appearance?
- Changes in sensation?
- Other physical problems?

How are you going to solve these problems? What options are available?

- Bladder retraining
- Pelvic floor physical therapy
- Acupuncture, Massage, Other Alternative Therapies
- Medications
- Surgery
- Other

Where will you get support?
- Local cancer support groups
- Post-cancer care programs
- Online or virtual support options
- Local places of worship
- Other

Where will your caregiver get support?
- Local support groups for caregivers
- Home care agencies
- Online or virtual support options
- Local places of worship
- Other

Post-surgery Tips (First 4-6 Weeks)
- Buy continence briefs and pads (maximum absorbency) to have ready at home
- Buy puppy pads for extra nighttime leakage protection
- Bladder retraining activities:
    - decrease overall caffeine intake to 1 drink per day
    - stay hydrated throughout the day—water is best

- o   NO alcohol the first 4-6 weeks after surgery
- o   avoid or minimize consumption of common bladder irritants: alcohol, caffeine, carbonated beverages, MSG, citrus, spicy foods
- o   schedule times to void
  - ▪   start with every hour
  - ▪   increase this time by 10 minutes/day if possible
  - ▪   work up to voiding every 2 hours (eventual goal is voiding every 3-4 hours)
- Be aware of what to expect in regaining urinary control as you recover
- Begin pelvic floor strengthening exercises as soon as possible (check with your surgeon first). See Chapter 7 for details on doing Kegels the correct way

Bladder Healthy Habits Guideline

These tips are included throughout your Progress Checkpoints. They are for the long-term; following them as part of your daily routine will help ensure a healthier, happier bladder.

Adequate Fluid Intake
- Drink 6-8 glasses of liquid daily (not caffeinated). Aim for half your body weight in ounces
- Drink throughout the day, less frequently at night before bedtime
- Avoid soda/pop (even sugar-free)

Eliminate (or reduce) Bladder Irritants
- Food and drinks that irritate bladder and can increase urine output:
  - o   Caffeinated drinks (coffee, tea, soda/pop)
  - o   Carbonated drinks (soda/pop, sparkling water or juice)

- o Alcohol
- o Chocolate
- o Citrus
- o Artificial Sweeteners
- o MSG (Monosodium Glutamate)

No "JIC"-ing!

"I'll use the toilet 'Just In Case'"—this can make for a fussy, unpredictable bladder! Try to wait until you sense the first urge to urinate, then if you can, let that urge pass (your bladder is only half-full at the first urge). This helps to retrain the bladder to go on a more normal schedule, reducing urgency/frequency problems.

Do Pelvic Floor Exercises Daily as prescribed by your physical therapist, or as suggested in this book

Practice Relaxation/Meditation Daily

This is good to help your body deal with stress and keep your bladder muscles calm.

- Diaphragmatic breathing
- Yoga or Chair Yoga
- Meditation or Prayer
- Journaling
- Other: Get creative!

Keep moving!

Stay as active as you possibly can, whether you walk, use a cane, or use a wheelchair.

Bladder Function Baseline Assessment

You'll find this assessment included in each of the two baseline checks in the Progress Notes.

Bladder Function Basics (Normal)

1. Bladder capacity = 300-400 ml, or about 16 oz. (the size of a Grande Latte)
2. 8 voids per day, 1 or less at night (1-2 voids/night if you're over age 65)
3. Voids are every 3-4 hours
4. Urine stream is strong, continuous (no stop-start)
5. Urine is clear or light straw-colored
6. Urine stream should stop completely with no dribbling afterward
7. Voiding is not painful
8. Urge to void sensation is present

Breathing

- How much are you holding your breath? Is it a habit that needs correcting?
- Balls Breathing: an easy way to get your pelvic floor working with your breathing muscle. This helps the pelvic floor work with your diaphragm (breathing muscle) and with your abdominal muscles.
  Remember the cue? *"Breathe Deep Into Your Balls"* (page 34).
  - Start practicing Balls Breathing for 5 breath cycles at first. A "breath cycle" is one breath in and one breath out. Don't try to hurry through this, allow the breaths to be at a slower pace. Gradually work up to 10 breath cycles at a time. Practice this "reconnection" exercise 3 times a day.

Leakage Baseline Self-Assessment

You'll find this assessment included in each baseline check as well as each Progress Check Point.

Urgency Incontinence or Urgency / Frequency Fix-It Tips

The Six Urge Suppression Strategies (summary only; refer back to Chapter 5 for details):

1. Stay still, don't panic
2. Deep breathing
3. Pelvic floor contractions
4. Distraction (includes Square Breathing)
5. Pressure on perineal area
6. Toe Taps

Practice them as needed when that strong urge hits. Try each one of them for at least one day, one strategy per day. Pick the two strategies that work best and use them consistently.

You can chart your progress with these strategies in the Progress Notes section.

Kegels Done Right

These exercises are also referred to as Pelvic Floor Contractions.

You need to do both Slow Holds and Quick Flicks for best results (instructions below).

Slow Holds: to retrain the slow-twitch endurance muscle fibers of the pelvic floor

- ✓ Tighten/flex pelvic floor muscles. Focus on the front part of the pelvic floor under the scrotum and penis.
- ✓ Try one of the cues below to get the right movement:
  - o pretend to stop the flow of urine
  - o "pull the turtle's head into its shell" (the turtle's head = your penis)
  - o "nuts to guts" (draw your testicles upward toward your belly)
- ✓ Make sure to relax the muscles between contractions!
- ✓ Start with what you can! Most guys can only do about 3 contractions at first before the muscles tire out! If that's all you can do, then 3 is your baseline starting point. Work up from there, until you can do 10 contractions.
- ✓ Gradually increase the time you can hold the contraction:
  - ▪ Hold times = 1 second → 3 seconds → 5 seconds → 10 seconds
- ✓ If you can do 6 sets of 10 contractions, without breath-holding and without muscle fatigue, then you can move up to the next hold time. (6 sets of 10 contractions = 60 contractions total per day)
- ✓ Do your 6 sets throughout the day, some in the morning, some mid-day, some in the evening.
- ✓ **STOP the exercise if you feel pain in the penis, perineal area, or rectum, or if you experience dizziness or light headedness. You might be overdoing it. Take a break, then go back to doing less repetitions or holding it for less time. If these symptoms persist, contact your physician.

"Quick Flicks": to retrain the fast-twitch power and speed muscle fibers.

➢ Contract/flex pelvic floor muscles strong and fast (1 second or less). No cheating from your nearby muscles (butt, inner thighs, low back)!

➢ Keep breathing as you do your quick flicks. No need to coordinate these with the exhale.

➢ General recommendation: start with 6 sets of 5 contractions, gradually build up the number of contractions (reps) until you can do 6 sets of 10 quick flicks correctly without muscle fatigue.

   o 6 sets of 5 contractions = 30 total
   o 6 sets of 10 contractions = 60 total

➢ Do sets throughout the day, some in morning, some mid-day, some in evening.

➢ **STOP the exercise if you feel pain in the penis, perineal area, or rectum, or if you experience dizziness or light headedness. You might be overdoing it or using too much force. Take a break, then go back to doing less repetitions or contracting with less effort. If these symptoms persist, contact your physician.

Checking Your Technique: if you're doing your Kegels correctly:
→ You can feel the contraction below base of the penis and scrotum
→ Testicles should rise and penis should retract slightly
→ Lower abdominal muscles pull in, not bulge out or downward
→ Inner thighs, buttocks, and upper abdominal muscles should not clench or tighten
→ You are not holding your breath
→ Movement of pelvic floor muscles is subtle. You're not doing a max bench press or squat. Don't try to squeeze with all your might.

You can track your personal progress with these exercises in the Progress Notes section / Checkpoints.

Stress Incontinence Fix-It Tips and Strategies

- **Breathing:** Avoid holding your breath! Especially when changing positions or lifting
- **EXhale with EXertion**. Remember to exhale (breathe out) when:
    - sitting up in bed
    - going from sitting to standing position
    - lifting an object, especially from floor level
    - pushing or pulling a heavy door or other object
- Practice your pelvic floor contraction exercises (**Kegels Done Right**) daily.

Pad Graduating Protocol "Ditch The Depends"
(created by Jo Milios, PhD)
1. Wear full briefs day + night
2. Graduate to wearing maximum strength pads day + night
3. Minimal leakage at night? Graduate to wearing a shield at night
4. Shields dry for three nights in a row? Ditch them!
5. Wait 5 minutes to apply pad in the morning. Increase wait time by 5 minutes a day.
6. Continue to wear pad, with less thickness, during the day when at home. Change to thicker pad when going out of the house or when doing more strenuous activity.
7. Reduce to minimal thickness pad during the day. Continue with no pads or shields at night.
8. Remove pad before bedtime, gradually increasing the time between pad removal and bedtime.
9. Reduce to a guard or shield for daytime use. Continue to increase time in the morning and in the evening without the guard.
10. Reduce to wearing NO pad during the day. Place a small shield in your pocket "just in case."
11. Forget that the shield is in your pocket? You are DRY!

Plan for Long-Term Success: Fitting It into Your Life

These tips will also be included in your Progress Notes Checkpoints.

✓ **Habit Stacking**
  - List three habits you do already to stack Kegels Plus exercises onto (slow + quick):
  - List three habits you do already to stack Balls Breathing onto:
  - List three movements you do already that you can add a pelvic floor contraction to (e.g., squats, bridges, lifting anything, etc.):

✓ **Reminders and Prompts**
  - How will you remember to stay consistent? What prompts can you use?
  - List at least three ways:

✓ **Accountability**
  - Do you plan to seek out an accountability buddy? Who is it?
  - In person, virtual, or combination of both?
  - How often and when will you meet?

✓ **Consistency**
  - For best recovery results, exercises and strategies need to be practiced DAILY.
  - If returning to exercise, begin with 2-3 days/week, then work up from there.
  - If you miss a day or two, just press "restart" and pick up where you left off.

PISS OFF (Literally)

PROGRESS NOTES

Chart Your Progress Step-By-Step

In this section, you can track your progress week-by-week, or at whatever intervals you choose. I've set up one example of a progress timeline that you can follow.

Tracking your progress can be very helpful and motivating. It provides objective proof that you are getting better, even if you feel far away from your goal. Below you will see a sample timeline, which includes the prehab phase. If you've already had your surgery, you can omit this part.

5 weeks before surgery → SURGERY →
— 2 weeks — 4 weeks — 8 weeks — 12 weeks — 16 weeks post-surgery

When to do Baseline Checks:
—5 weeks before surgery date, if possible
—After catheter removal post-surgery (with clearance from your surgeon)

Baseline Checks include:
—Bladder Function Baseline Assessment
—Leakage Baseline Self-Assessment

When to do Progress Checks (suggested):
—2 weeks, 4 weeks, 8 weeks, 12 weeks, and 16 weeks post-surgery
—You can do weekly checks if you'd prefer.
—Keep the end goal in mind! Some weeks you will notice more progress than others, some weeks you may seem to regress and get worse. This is normal as you recover. What's important is that your leakage reduces overall from start to finish. There will be a few bumps along the way. Expect them. Also expect to move past them.

You'll find each Progress "Check Point" listed on the next pages, with accompanying tools and measures.

These are based off the three steps of the Kegels Plus approach:

1) Pay Attention to your pelvic floor
2) Pelvic Floor working with rest of body = Teamwork
3) Plan for long term success = fit this into the flow of your life

Ready to get started?

PROGRESS NOTES

PREHAB PHASE (5 weeks before surgery)   Date _____

Pre-Surgery Baseline Check #1. Your Bladder Function Baseline

1. Bladder capacity: how much am I voiding when I urinate?
(You can measure it or estimate: small, medium, or large amount)
2. How many times do I urinate during the day? _____ During the night? _____
3. How long do I go in between voids? _____hours, or _____ minutes
4. How's my urine stream? Circle one answer in each pair below.

> Strong   weak/slow
>
> Continuous   stop-start
>
> Starts right away   hesitates

5. Does my urine stream stop completely when done? Is there dribbling afterward?
6. Is my urine clear or light straw-colored? Is it dark yellow, brownish, or cloudy? Is it blood-tinged?
7. Do I have pain with urination?
8. Can I feel a sensation of urge to urinate?
9. Can I delay that first urge sensation for at least 15-20 minutes?

Compare your results with the Normal Bladder Function Basics on page 130 of the Toolkit. Write your answers below.

How close is your baseline to normal?

Where does it fall short? What needs improvement?

Pre-Surgery Questions Checklist (pages 126): Bring this to your surgical consult appointment.

Post-Surgery Tips (pages 127-128): Review these now; begin them on Day 1 after your surgery.

Pre-Surgery Baseline Check# 2. Your Leakage Baseline
**NOTE: only do this one if you are experiencing some incontinence prior to surgery

LEAKAGE BASELINE SELF-ASSESSMENT

1. On a scale of 0-10, how bad is your leakage now? (0=none, 10=worst ever). Circle your answer.

$$0 - 1 - 2 - 3 - 4 - 5 - 6 - 7 - 8 - 9 - 10$$

2. How often do you usually experience leakage?   (circle your answer)
3 times/week or less
Once a day
At least 3 times/day
More than 3x/day
I've lost count it happens so much!

3. How many times are you getting up at night to urinate?
(circle your answer)
None
1-2 times
3-4 times
5 or more times

PROGRESS NOTES

4. What things trigger your leakage?   (circle your answer)

Sneezing, coughing, or laughing
Exercise or lifting heavier objects
Changing positions (sitting to standing, lying down to sitting up, etc)
Running water, proximity to garage door, front door, or bathroom
Strong urge to urinate
Nothing--it just happens without warning
Other:

5. What kind of protection do you need to wear?   (circle your answer)
Nothing
Shield
Guard or pad
Full protection briefs/pullups

6. How many briefs/pads are you going through during the day? _____

7. How many briefs/pads are you going through at night? _____

8. How full are your briefs or pads when you change them?
(circle your answer)
A few drops
Wet but not to the edges
Wet to the edges/sides
Totally soaked

9. What time of day do you notice the most leakage?

(circle your answer)
Nighttime
Morning
Afternoon
Evening
Can't tell, it's all the time

10. How long can you delay the need to urinate?   (circle your answer)
More than one hour
30-60 minutes
15 minutes
3-5 minutes
Less than one minute
Other:

11. If you had to live with your incontinence the way it is now, what would that be like?   (circle your answer)
I'd be satisfied
Inconvenient but I could live with it
Frustrating
Terrible

PROGRESS NOTES

AFTER SURGERY AND CATHETER REMOVAL   Date _____

Post-Surgery Tips (page 127-128): Begin these now, continue for the first 4-6 weeks after surgery

Post-Surgery Baseline Check #1. Your Bladder Function Baseline

1. Bladder capacity: how much am I voiding when I urinate?
(You can measure it or estimate: small, medium, or large amount)
2. How many times do I urinate during the day? _____ During the night? _____
3. How long do I go in between voids? ____hours, or _____ minutes
4. How's my urine stream? Circle one answer in each pair below.

       Strong weak/slow

       Continuous stop-start

       Starts right away hesitates
5. Does my urine stream stop completely when done? Is there dribbling afterward?
6. Is my urine clear or light straw-colored? Is it dark yellow, brownish, or cloudy? Is it blood-tinged?
7. Do I have pain with urination?
8. Can I feel a sensation of urge to urinate?
9. Can I delay that first urge sensation for at least 15-20 minutes?

Compare your results with the **Normal Bladder Function Basics** in the Recovery Toolkit, page 130. Write your answers below.

How close is your baseline to normal?

Where does it fall short? What needs improvement?

Post-Surgery Baseline Check #2. Your Leakage Baseline

LEAKAGE BASELINE SELF-ASSESSMENT

1. On a scale of 0-10, how bad is your leakage now? (0=none, 10=worst ever). Circle your answer.
      0 — 1 — 2 — 3 — 4 — 5 — 6 — 7 — 8 — 9 — 10

2. How often do you usually experience leakage? (circle your answer)
3 times/week or less
Once a day
At least 3 times/day
More than 3x/day
I've lost count it happens so much!

3. How many times are you getting up at night to urinate?
(circle your answer)
None
1-2 times
3-4 times
5 or more times

4. What things trigger your leakage? (circle your answer)
Sneezing, coughing, or laughing
Exercise or lifting heavier objects
Changing positions (sitting to standing, lying down to sitting up, etc.)
Running water, proximity to garage door, front door, or bathroom
Strong urge to urinate
Nothing--it just happens without warning

5. What kind of protection do you need to wear?   (circle your answer)

Nothing
Shield
Guard or pad
Full protection briefs/pullups

6. How many briefs/pads are you going through during the day?   _____

7. How many briefs/pads are you going through at night?   _____

8. How full are your briefs or pads when you change them?
(circle your answer)
A few drops
Wet but not to the edges
Wet to the edges/sides
Totally soaked

9. What time of day do you notice the most leakage?
(circle your answer)
Nighttime
Morning
Afternoon
Evening
Can't tell, it's all the time

10. How long can you delay the need to urinate?   (circle your answer)
More than one hour
30-60 minutes
15 minutes
3-5 minutes
Less than one minute

11. If you had to live with your incontinence the way it is now, what would that be like?   (circle answer)

I'd be satisfied

Inconvenient but I could live with it

Frustrating

Terrible

NOTES

PROGRESS NOTES
WEEK 2 AFTER SURGERY   Date _____

Kegels Plus Checkpoints
1. PAY ATTENTION
Breathing (page 130):
> Breath-holding: always? Sometimes? Rarely? (circle one)
> Practice Balls Breathing: for _____ breath cycles, _____times/day

Urgency Incontinence or Urgency/Frequency Check: (if applicable; see page 131 for details)
What urge suppression strategies work best for me? Pick the top 2.
> 1. _____
> 2. _____

How many times am I getting up at night to use the bathroom? _____
How long can I now "hold back the tide" when I get the urge? _____ minutes

Is the urge less intense and less frequent? Yes   No

NOTE: the goal is not to hold it so long that you are miserable. Try gradually increasing your hold time. Even one minute per week is good progress. "Normal" hold time is about 20 minutes.

Kegels Done Right: (i.e., Pelvic Floor Contractions), pages 131-133
Slow Hold Contractions: can do _____ sets, _____ reps, _____-second hold each rep
Quick Flick Contractions: can do ___ sets, ___ reps
Position I'm doing exercises: ___lying down ___ sitting ___ standing

--How's my technique? Go through the checklist on page 133

147

2. TEAMWORK (Pelvic Floor Working With Rest of Body)

Do I EXhale with Exertion? (page 134)
___ never   ___ sometimes   ___ still have to think about it   ___ it's almost second nature

Other Physical Activity or Exercise I'm Doing:
My Activity is: _____
How often? ____ days/week   For how long? _____ minutes/each time

3. FIT IT INTO YOUR LIFE (Have a Plan for Long-Term Success)

Post-Surgery Tips (pages 127-128): Continue following these for first 4-6 weeks after surgery

Pad Graduation Protocol (page 134) :
Which step am I on now? Step ___
What's my goal for next check point? Step ___

Move With Purpose (page 135):
Habit Stacking
What activities can I fit my Balls Breathing into? (list three)

What activities or movements can I fit my Kegels into? (list three)

Reminders
What reminders can I use to stay consistent? (list three)

Consistency
I'm sticking with my Action Plan ____ days/week

Accountability

Do I have an accountability buddy?

Have I checked in with them during this Check Point time?

When is my next meeting day/time?

LEAKAGE SELF-ASSESSMENT, Week 2

1. On a scale of 0-10, how bad is your leakage now? (0=none, 10=worst ever). Circle your answer.

   0 — 1 — 2 — 3 — 4 — 5 — 6 — 7 — 8 — 9 — 10

2. How often do you usually experience leakage?   (circle your answer)

Once a day

At least 3 times/day

More than 3x/day

I've lost count it happens so much!

3. How many times are you getting up at night to urinate?

None

1-2 times

3-4 times

5 or more times

4. What things trigger your leakage?

Sneezing, coughing, or laughing

Exercise or lifting heavier objects

Changing positions (sitting to standing, lying down to sitting up, etc)

Running water, proximity to garage door, front door, or bathroom

Strong urge to urinate

Nothing--it just happens without warning

5. What kind of protection do you need to wear?
Nothing
Shield
Guard or pad
Full protection briefs/pullups

6. How many briefs/pads are you going through during the day? _____

7. How many briefs/pads are you going through at night? _____

8. How full are your briefs or pads when you change them?
A few drops
Wet but not to the edges
Wet to the edges/sides
Totally soaked

9. What time of day do you notice the most leakage?
Nighttime
Morning
Afternoon
Evening
Can't tell, it's all the time

10. How long can you delay the need to urinate?
More than one hour
30-60 minutes
15 minutes
3-5 minutes
Less than one minute

PROGRESS NOTES
WEEK 4 AFTER SURGERY   Date _____

Kegels Plus Checkpoints
1. PAY ATTENTION
Breathing (page 130):
    Breath-holding: always? Sometimes? Rarely? (circle one)
    Practice Balls Breathing: for _____ breath cycles, _____times/day

Urgency Incontinence or Urgency/Frequency Check: (if applicable; see page 131 for details)
What urge suppression strategies work best for me? Pick the top 2.
    1. _____
    2. _____
How many times am I getting up at night to use the bathroom? _____
How long can I now "hold back the tide" when I get the urge? _____ minutes
Is the urge less intense and less frequent? Yes   No

NOTE: the goal is not to hold it so long that you are miserable. Try gradually increasing your hold time. Even one minute per week is good progress. "Normal" hold time is about 20 minutes.

Kegels Done Right: (i.e., Pelvic Floor Contractions), pages 131-133
    Slow Hold Contractions: can do _____ sets, _____ reps, _____-second hold each rep
    Quick Flick Contractions: can do ___ sets, ___ reps
    Position I'm doing exercises: ___lying down ___ sitting ___ standing

--How's my technique? Go through the checklist on page 133

2. TEAMWORK (Pelvic Floor Working With Rest of Body)

Do I EXhale with Exertion? (page 134)
___ never   ___ sometimes   ___ still have to think about it   ___ it's almost second nature

Other Physical Activity or Exercise I'm Doing:
My Activity is: _____
How often? ____ days/week   For how long? _____ minutes/each time

3. FIT IT INTO YOUR LIFE (Have a Plan for Long-Term Success)

Post-Surgery Tips (pages 127-128): Continue following these for first 4-6 weeks after surgery

Pad Graduation Protocol (page 134) :
Which step am I on now? Step ___
What's my goal for next check point? Step ___

<u>Move With Purpose (page 135):</u>
Habit Stacking
What activities can I fit my Balls Breathing into? (list three)

What activities or movements can I fit my Kegels into? (list three)

Reminders
What reminders can I use to stay consistent? (list three)

Consistency
I'm sticking with my Action Plan ____ days/week

Accountability
Do I have an accountability buddy?
Have I checked in with them during this Check Point time?
When is my next meeting day/time?

LEAKAGE SELF-ASSESSMENT, Week 4

1. On a scale of 0-10, how bad is your leakage now? (0=none, 10=worst ever). Circle your answer.

     0 — 1 — 2 — 3 — 4 — 5 — 6 — 7 — 8 — 9 — 10

2. How often do you usually experience leakage? (circle your answer)
Once a day
At least 3 times/day
More than 3x/day
I've lost count it happens so much!

3. How many times are you getting up at night to urinate?
None
1-2 times
3-4 times
5 or more times

4. What things trigger your leakage?
Sneezing, coughing, or laughing
Exercise or lifting heavier objects
Changing positions (sitting to standing, lying down to sitting up, etc)
Running water, proximity to garage door, front door, or bathroom
Strong urge to urinate
Nothing--it just happens without warning

5. What kind of protection do you need to wear?
Nothing
Shield
Guard or pad
Full protection briefs/pullups

6. How many briefs/pads are you going through during the day? _____

7. How many briefs/pads are you going through at night? _____

8. How full are your briefs or pads when you change them?
A few drops
Wet but not to the edges
Wet to the edges/sides
Totally soaked

9. What time of day do you notice the most leakage?
Nighttime
Morning
Afternoon
Evening
Can't tell, it's all the time

10. How long can you delay the need to urinate?
More than one hour
30-60 minutes
15 minutes
3-5 minutes
Less than one minute

PROGRESS NOTES
WEEK 8 AFTER SURGERY   Date _____

Kegels Plus Checkpoints
1. PAY ATTENTION
Breathing (page 130):
    Breath-holding: always? Sometimes? Rarely? (circle one)
    Practice Balls Breathing: for _____ breath cycles, _____times/day

Urgency Incontinence or Urgency/Frequency Check: (if applicable; see page 131 for details)
What urge suppression strategies work best for me? Pick the top 2.
    1. _____
    2. _____
How many times am I getting up at night to use the bathroom? _____
How long can I now "hold back the tide" when I get the urge? _____ minutes
Is the urge less intense and less frequent? Yes   No

NOTE: the goal is not to hold it so long that you are miserable. Try gradually increasing your hold time. Even one minute per week is good progress. "Normal" hold time is about 20 minutes.

Kegels Done Right: (i.e., Pelvic Floor Contractions), pages 131-133
Slow Hold Contractions: can do _____ sets, _____ reps, _____-second hold each rep
Quick Flick Contractions: can do ___ sets, ___ reps
Position I'm doing exercises: ___lying down ___ sitting ___ standing

--How's my technique? Go through the checklist on page 133

2. TEAMWORK (Pelvic Floor Working With Rest of Body)

Do I EXhale with Exertion? (page 134)
___ never   ___ sometimes   ___still have to think about it   ___ it's almost second nature

Other Physical Activity or Exercise I'm Doing:
My Activity is: _____
How often? ____ days/week   For how long? _____ minutes/each time

3. FIT IT INTO YOUR LIFE (Have a Plan for Long-Term Success)

Post-Surgery Tips (pages 127-128): Continue following these for first 4-6 weeks after surgery

Pad Graduation Protocol (page 134) :
Which step am I on now? Step ___
What's my goal for next check point? Step ___

Move With Purpose (page 135):
Habit Stacking
What activities can I fit my Balls Breathing into? (list three)

What activities or movements can I fit my Kegels into? (list three)

Reminders
What reminders can I use to stay consistent? (list three)

Consistency
I'm sticking with my Action Plan ____ days/week

Accountability

Do I have an accountability buddy?

Have I checked in with them during this Check Point time?

When is my next meeting day/time?

LEAKAGE SELF-ASSESSMENT, Week 8

1. On a scale of 0-10, how bad is your leakage now? (0=none, 10=worst ever). Circle your answer.

$$0 — 1 — 2 — 3 — 4 — 5 — 6 — 7 — 8 — 9 — 10$$

2. How often do you usually experience leakage? (circle your answer)

Once a day

At least 3 times/day

More than 3x/day

I've lost count it happens so much!

3. How many times are you getting up at night to urinate?

None

1-2 times

3-4 times

5 or more times

4. What things trigger your leakage?

Sneezing, coughing, or laughing

Exercise or lifting heavier objects

Changing positions (sitting to standing, lying down to sitting up, etc)

Running water, proximity to garage door, front door, or bathroom

Strong urge to urinate

Nothing--it just happens without warning

5. What kind of protection do you need to wear?
Nothing
Shield
Guard or pad
Full protection briefs/pullups

6. How many briefs/pads are you going through during the day?   _____

7. How many briefs/pads are you going through at night?   _____

8. How full are your briefs or pads when you change them?
A few drops
Wet but not to the edges
Wet to the edges/sides
Totally soaked

9. What time of day do you notice the most leakage?
Nighttime
Morning
Afternoon
Evening
Can't tell, it's all the time

10. How long can you delay the need to urinate?
More than one hour
30-60 minutes
15 minutes
3-5 minutes
Less than one minute

PROGRESS NOTES
WEEK 12 AFTER SURGERY   Date _____

Kegels Plus Checkpoints
1. PAY ATTENTION
Breathing (page 130):
 Breath-holding: always? Sometimes? Rarely? (circle one)
 Practice Balls Breathing: for _____ breath cycles, _____times/day

Urgency Incontinence or Urgency/Frequency Check: (if applicable; see page 131 for details)
What urge suppression strategies work best for me? Pick the top 2.
 1. _____
 2. _____
How many times am I getting up at night to use the bathroom? _____
How long can I now "hold back the tide" when I get the urge? _____ minutes
Is the urge less intense and less frequent? Yes   No

NOTE: the goal is not to hold it so long that you are miserable. Try gradually increasing your hold time. Even one minute per week is good progress. "Normal" hold time is about 20 minutes.

Kegels Done Right: (i.e., Pelvic Floor Contractions), pages 131-133
 Slow Hold Contractions: can do ____ sets, ____ reps, ____-second hold each rep
 Quick Flick Contractions: can do ___ sets, ___ reps
 Position I'm doing exercises: ___lying down ___ sitting ___ standing

--How's my technique? Go through the checklist on page 133

2. TEAMWORK (Pelvic Floor Working With Rest of Body)

Do I EXhale with Exertion? (page 134)
___ never   ___ sometimes   ___still have to think about it   ___ it's almost second nature

Other Physical Activity or Exercise I'm Doing:
My Activity is: _____
How often? ____ days/week   For how long? _____ minutes/each time

3. FIT IT INTO YOUR LIFE (Have a Plan for Long-Term Success)

Post-Surgery Tips (pages 127-128): Continue following these for first 4-6 weeks after surgery

Pad Graduation Protocol (page 134) :
Which step am I on now? Step ___
What's my goal for next check point? Step ___

Move With Purpose (page 135):
Habit Stacking
What activities can I fit my Balls Breathing into? (list three)

What activities or movements can I fit my Kegels into? (list three)

Reminders
What reminders can I use to stay consistent? (list three)

Consistency
I'm sticking with my Action Plan ____ days/week

Accountability

Do I have an accountability buddy?

Have I checked in with them during this Check Point time?

When is my next meeting day/time?

LEAKAGE SELF-ASSESSMENT, Week 12

1. On a scale of 0-10, how bad is your leakage now? (0=none, 10=worst ever). Circle your answer.

    0 — 1 — 2 — 3 — 4 — 5 — 6 — 7 — 8 — 9 — 10

2. How often do you usually experience leakage?   (circle your answer)

Once a day

At least 3 times/day

More than 3x/day

I've lost count it happens so much!

3. How many times are you getting up at night to urinate?

None

1-2 times

3-4 times

5 or more times

4. What things trigger your leakage?

Sneezing, coughing, or laughing

Exercise or lifting heavier objects

Changing positions (sitting to standing, lying down to sitting up, etc)

Running water, proximity to garage door, front door, or bathroom

Strong urge to urinate

Nothing--it just happens without warning

5. What kind of protection do you need to wear?
Nothing
Shield
Guard or pad
Full protection briefs/pullups

6. How many briefs/pads are you going through during the day? _____

7. How many briefs/pads are you going through at night? _____

8. How full are your briefs or pads when you change them?
A few drops
Wet but not to the edges
Wet to the edges/sides
Totally soaked

9. What time of day do you notice the most leakage?
Nighttime
Morning
Afternoon
Evening
Can't tell, it's all the time

10. How long can you delay the need to urinate?
More than one hour
30-60 minutes
15 minutes
3-5 minutes
Less than one minute

PROGRESS NOTES
WEEK 16 AFTER SURGERY   Date _____

Kegels Plus Checkpoints
1. PAY ATTENTION
Breathing (page 130):
    Breath-holding: always? Sometimes? Rarely? (circle one)
    Practice Balls Breathing: for _____ breath cycles, _____times/day

Urgency Incontinence or Urgency/Frequency Check: (if applicable; see page 131 for details)
What urge suppression strategies work best for me? Pick the top 2.
    1. _____
    2. _____
How many times am I getting up at night to use the bathroom? _____
How long can I now "hold back the tide" when I get the urge? _____ minutes
Is the urge less intense and less frequent? Yes   No

NOTE: the goal is not to hold it so long that you are miserable. Try gradually increasing your hold time. Even one minute per week is good progress. "Normal" hold time is about 20 minutes.

Kegels Done Right: (i.e., Pelvic Floor Contractions), pages 131-133
Slow Hold Contractions: can do ____ sets, ____ reps, ____-second hold each rep
Quick Flick Contractions: can do ___ sets, ___ reps
Position I'm doing exercises: ___lying down ___ sitting ___ standing

--How's my technique? Go through the checklist on page 133

2. TEAMWORK (Pelvic Floor Working With Rest of Body)

Do I EXhale with Exertion? (page 134)
___ never   ___ sometimes   ___still have to think about it   ___ it's almost second nature

Other Physical Activity or Exercise I'm Doing:
My Activity is: _____
How often? ____ days/week   For how long? _____ minutes/each time

3. FIT IT INTO YOUR LIFE (Have a Plan for Long-Term Success)

Post-Surgery Tips (pages 127-128): Continue following these for first 4-6 weeks after surgery

Pad Graduation Protocol (page 134) :
Which step am I on now? Step ___
What's my goal for next check point? Step ___

Move With Purpose (page 135):
Habit Stacking
What activities can I fit my Balls Breathing into? (list three)

What activities or movements can I fit my Kegels into? (list three)

Reminders
What reminders can I use to stay consistent? (list three)

Consistency
I'm sticking with my Action Plan ____ days/week

PROGRESS NOTES

Accountability
Do I have an accountability buddy?
Have I checked in with them during this Check Point time?
When is my next meeting day/time?

LEAKAGE SELF-ASSESSMENT, Week 16

1. On a scale of 0-10, how bad is your leakage now? (0=none, 10=worst ever). Circle your answer.
     0 — 1 — 2 — 3 — 4 — 5 — 6 — 7 — 8 — 9 — 10

2. How often do you usually experience leakage?   (circle your answer)
Once a day
At least 3 times/day
More than 3x/day
I've lost count it happens so much!

3. How many times are you getting up at night to urinate?
None
1-2 times
3-4 times
5 or more times

4. What things trigger your leakage?
Sneezing, coughing, or laughing
Exercise or lifting heavier objects
Changing positions (sitting to standing, lying down to sitting up, etc)
Running water, proximity to garage door, front door, or bathroom
Strong urge to urinate
Nothing--it just happens without warning

5. What kind of protection do you need to wear?
Nothing
Shield
Guard or pad
Full protection briefs/pullups

6. How many briefs/pads are you going through during the day? _____

7. How many briefs/pads are you going through at night? _____

8. How full are your briefs or pads when you change them?
A few drops
Wet but not to the edges
Wet to the edges/sides
Totally soaked

9. What time of day do you notice the most leakage?
Nighttime
Morning
Afternoon
Evening
Can't tell, it's all the time

10. How long can you delay the need to urinate?
More than one hour
30-60 minutes
15 minutes
3-5 minutes
Less than one minute

11. If you had to live with your incontinence the way it is now, what would that be like?   (circle answer)

I'd be satisfied

Inconvenient but I could live with it

Frustrating

Terrible

NOTES, TAKEAWAYS:

Did you reach your goal for your Action Plan?

If so, congratulations! I hope you have found this book helpful in getting your bladder control back.

If you haven't yet reached your goal, keep going. Not everyone succeeds 100% within 12 or 16 weeks.

Most likely you have seen some progress in your bladder control since you started your Action Plan. Keep working at it.

If you've struggled with this, perhaps it would be good to seek out some professional guidance from a qualified pelvic floor physical therapist or exercise/fitness professional. They may be able to help you fill in the gaps and get you to where you want to be.

This is an Action Plan for life now! By maintaining good pelvic floor strength and healthy bladder habits, you can keep control over your bladder so that it no longer controls you. The only way to maintain this is to work your pelvic floor muscles through exercise and other activities. Fit it into your daily activities, and this will be much easier to do long-term.

I wish you the best of luck as you get back to enjoying life!

Laura McKaig

NOTES

NOTES

ABOUT THE AUTHOR

Laura McKaig is a licensed physical therapist in the U.S. with nearly 20 years of clinical experience. *(Her journey into the pelvic health specialty has had a unique path, which she shares in this book.)* She owns and operates Laura McKaig Physical Therapy LLC, in Olathe, Kansas, and is one of the few clinicians in the Kansas City area specializing exclusively in pelvic floor physical therapy for men as well as women. Laura is an outspoken advocate for men's health and for prostate cancer rehabilitation, writing publications, teaching classes, and volunteering with local and national prostate cancer groups. She has also advocated on Capitol Hill in Washington, D.C. for legislation supporting prostate cancer patients and survivors.

Bio Photo Credit: Cory Finley, Seven Images, KC

BIBLIOGRAPHY

Chang, Peter, Andrew A. Wagner, Meredith M. Regan, Joseph A. Smith, Christopher S. Saigal, Mark S. Litwin, Jim C. Hu et al. "Prospective multicenter comparison of open and robotic radical prostatectomy: The PROST-QA/RP2 Consortium." *The Journal of Urology* 207, no. 1 (2022): 127-136.

Dr. Joanne Milios' Pad Weaning Protocol. Dr. Jo Milios (PhD) MACP B.Sci (Physiotherapy) Western Australia

Filocamo, Maria Teresa, Vincenzo Li Marzi, Giulio Del Popolo, Filippo Cecconi, Michele Marzocco, Aldo Tosto, and Giulio Nicita. "Effectiveness of early pelvic floor rehabilitation treatment for post-prostatectomy incontinence." *European Urology* 48, no. 5 (2005): 734-738.

Hodges, Paul W., Ryan E. Stafford, Leanne Hall, Patricia Neumann, Shan Morrison, Helena Frawley, Stuart Doorbar-Baptist et al. "Reconsideration of pelvic floor muscle training to prevent and treat incontinence after radical prostatectomy." In *Urologic Oncology: Seminars and Original Investigations*, vol. 38, no. 5, pp. 354-371. Elsevier, 2020.

Kaushik, Dharam, Pankil K. Shah, Neelam Mukherjee, Niannian Ji, Furkan Dursun, Addanki P. Kumar, Ian M. Thompson Jr et al. "Effects of yoga in men with prostate cancer on quality of life and immune response: a pilot randomized controlled trial." *Prostate Cancer and Prostatic Diseases* 25, no. 3 (2022): 531-538.

Kegel, Arnold H. "Progressive resistance exercise in the functional restoration of the perineal muscles." *American Journal of Obstetrics and Gynecology* 56, no. 2 (1948): 238-248.

Lopez, Pedro, Dennis R. Taaffe, Robert U. Newton, and Daniel A. Galvao. "Resistance exercise dosage in men with prostate cancer: systematic review, meta-analysis, and meta-regression." *Medicine and Science in Sports and Exercise* 53, no. 3 (2021): 459.

McGee, Robert W. "Tai Chi, Qigong and the Treatment of Cancer." *Biomedical Journal of Scientific & Technical Research* 34, no. 5 (2021): 27173-27182.

Milios, Joanne E., Timothy R. Ackland, and Daniel J. Green. "Pelvic floor muscle training in radical prostatectomy: a randomized controlled trial of the impacts on pelvic floor muscle function and urinary incontinence." *BMC Urology* 19, no. 1 (2019): 1-10.

Mungovan, Sean F., Sigrid V. Carlsson, Gregory C. Gass, Petra L. Graham, Jaspreet S. Sandhu, Oguz Akin, Peter T. Scardino, James A. Eastham, and Manish I. Patel. "Preoperative exercise interventions to optimize continence outcomes following radical prostatectomy." *Nature Reviews Urology* 18, no. 5 (2021): 259-281.

Schieszer, John. "Kegel Exercises After Prostate Surgery Called Into Question." Renal & Urology News. January 15, 2020. https://www.renalandurologynews.com/home/news/urology/prostate-cancer/kegel-exercises-after-prostate-surgery-called-into-question/.

Scott, Kelly M., Erika Gosai, Michelle H. Bradley, Steven Walton, Linda S. Hynan, Gary Lemack, and Claus Roehrborn. "Individualized pelvic physical therapy for the treatment of post-prostatectomy stress urinary incontinence and pelvic pain." *International Urology and Nephrology* 52 (2020): 655-659.

Siegel, A. "The Kegel Renaissance." *Journal of Urology and Research* 3, no. 4 (2016): 1061.

Winnall, Wendy. "A Pelvic Floor Exercise Program before Prostate Surgery Improves Urinary Continence." Prostate Cancer Foundation of Australia. December 3, 2019. https://www.pcfa.org.au/news-media/news/a-pelvic-floor-exercise-program-starting-before-prostate-surgery-improves-the-recovery-of-urinary-continence/.

Yang, Claire C. and Gerald W. Timm. "William E. Bradley and his contributions to urology." *The Journal of Urology* 179, no. 5 (2008): 1700-1703.

Made in the USA
Columbia, SC
02 March 2025